The Two Finger Diet

The Two Finger Diet

✦

How the Media Has Duped Women into Hating Themselves

Benjamin A Straight

iUniverse, Inc.
New York Lincoln Shanghai

The Two Finger Diet
How the Media Has Duped Women into Hating Themselves

iUniverse books may be ordered through booksellers or by contacting:

iUniverse
2021 Pine Lake Road, Suite 100
Lincoln, NE 68512
www.iuniverse.com
1-800-Authors (1-800-288-4677)

ISBN: 0-595-35017-8

Printed in the United States of America

Contents

The Two Finger Diet: How the Media Has Duped Women into Hating Themselves

I wrote this book between the fall of 2001 and the spring of 2003 while completing a Master's degree in Sociology. Much has changed since the completion of the writings, but I believe that the statistics, conclusions, and research are applicable for a number of years to come. I conducted and compiled this research in order to educate the American population about the forces at work to create the reality in which we all live. Ultimately, my goal is to educate women about the construction of the 'beauty image' as nothing more than an advertising scheme meant to sell commodities, and [hopefully] resulting from this will come an understanding that will reduce the societal repercussions such as eating disorders and cosmetic surgery.

I did not write this book to portray or to label women as victims of the advertising agencies. The responsibility for the 'beauty image' is not solely the advertisers. Women are not passive zombies acting purely out of advertisement brainwashing; we are all rational actors within society and are responsible for the decisions we make. I believe that the responsibility is shared and the fault with women is that they do not question the advertisements targeted at them by the media. However, I do believe that the advertisers create the reality to be consumed first and then women solidify the image by reproducing it and voting with their purchasing power. It then becomes a lived reality. I believe that, as a culture, we are too far into the matrix of this particular cultural mandate and constructed reality to question the originations of it or to ponder whether it is physically, mentally, and socially healthy. Basically, we accept the 'beauty image' as a cultural dictate that is expected by both men and women and we have for so long that we have forgotten that what we currently believe is not divine in nature nor permanent. The only thing constant is change.

Since I have finished this book, plastic surgery has skyrocketed in popularity. Numerous cable stations run reality television shows showing the daily routines of plastic surgeons and interviewing the women undergoing elective surgery.

According to the American Society of Aesthetic Plastic Surgery, nearly 8.3 million surgeries were conducted in 2003 which is a twenty percent increase over 2002, and the overall increase in cosmetic procedures has risen 293 percent since 1997 (www.surgery.org/press).

It is obvious that advertising influences us all, to some degree, whether we shun television or stay glued to it for hours. Because advertising is directed at different population segments (demographics) in order to increase sales, one could argue that groups that are heavily targeted with advertising would be more influenced by advertisements. A demographic group that has received notable attention from advertisers is women, primarily those between the ages of eighteen to thirty-four, women with children, and homemakers (Marchand 1985; Fiske 1989; Friedan 1963). I have noticed a disproportionate number of ads aimed at selling to women since my first awareness of advertisements in pre-adolescence. I also noticed that girls and young women were wearing the make-up and clothes that were mass-marketed. Not only that, but girls seemed to judge each other based on the new 'styles'; clothes and make-up could either destroy or bolster a girl's standing among her peers.

My interest continued through high school when I began learning about eating disorders and the theories of their origins. Both of my high schools that I attended taught that an eating disorder was a personal struggle for an individual to overcome. They further taught that the vast majority of eating disorders occurred in women. When questioned, most teachers stated that eating disorders stemmed from a feeling of inadequacy—mainly in terms of physical looks.

Researchers have found that unrealistic cultural expectations of thinness could be related to the prevalence of eating disorders among women (Garner et. al. 1980; Silverstein et. al. 1986; Bergeron and Senn 1998; Turner 1997). In fact, ninety percent of all anorexics are women (Druss and Henifin 1979). Because bulimia (practice of binging and purging) is practiced in secret, the actual incidence is unknown but researchers have found that as many as one-fifth of all high school and college age women display temporary bulimic symptoms (Sullivan et. al. 1996). Studies have been conducted on females in high school who frequently read beauty and health/fitness magazines (defined as at least once a month) and those who do not read these magazines. Gorrell reports that Steven Thomsen, Ph.D., found that "nearly 80 percent of frequent readers had induced vomiting, 73 percent had taken diet pills and 60 percent had used laxatives. And nearly two times as many women who limited their daily caloric intake also read health and fitness magazines more frequently compared with those who did not" (Gorrell 2001:24).

As I went through my undergraduate studies in college, I had more contact with women who had eating disorders both because of the close proximity of peers in residence halls (coed dormitories) and because of my job as a Resident Assistant [job where I oversaw the welfare of twenty-five to 240 students daily]. I had roommates and friends come to me for assistance in locating help for their friends with eating disorders. I was also a member of a social fraternity and spent all of my free time with the organization, which in turn spent most of its time with sororities. I learned of an informal and constant competition among females for reputation and status when I was exposed to sororities. Along with this competition came the feeling of inadequacy in regards to physical body structure and an attempt to maintain a thin body image. I had girlfriends who were members of sororities who told me what their 'sisters' would do in order to achieve the perceived physical standard and image set forth by their respective groups. I learned that these women had eating disorders, severe self-esteem issues, and other unhealthy personal habits.

I soon began to believe that the women I knew primarily judged other women in respect to body type and image. I also believed that the myth of women having to wear a certain product to attract a man came from advertising. This thought came to me while reading an issue of *Cosmopolitan* for a class I was taking.

I started thinking that there is a 'beauty myth' (Wolf 1991) that women were expected to live up to. My first thoughts were that this image came from advertising because I saw women (from an early age) reproducing the images that I had seen advertised; oddly, I never saw these images being perfectly replicated by women. I believe that the ideal projected by the 'beauty myth' is impossible to attain, even though people judge each other by this constantly changing standard. From this feeling of constant pressure to attain this image may come social problems such as eating disorders and an array of personal problems. The basis of advertising towards females is to make them feel bad [self-esteem] or guilty about not having a certain product. I want to study this topic in order to learn how capitalism has influenced the accepted standard of beauty and projected it to women through advertising, and how such ads manifest a negative reality individually that could aid in the construction of low self-esteem and eating disorders in women. I am further interested in how cosmetic surgery industry has become a multi-billion dollar industry since the 1980's and how this may be related to the construction of the modern 'beauty myth'. My goal is to present a number of opposing viewpoints and theories about how advertising, women's thought, and body practices interact (or are related).

In doing primary research on the topic, I first began viewing material on the subject in a Sociology class called Quantitative Research Methods. I learned of the method of research known as content analysis; this is integrated method, procedure, and technique for locating, identifying, retrieving, and analyzing documents for their relevance, significance, and meaning. The emphasis is on discovery and description, including search for contexts, underlying meanings, patterns, and processes (Altheide 1996). After researching and reading a [content analysis] methodology employed by prominent Sociologist Erving Goffman using ads containing females in submissive postures relative to men, I decided to use his model as a skeleton for part of my research. I used content analysis to find the frequency of coded phrases (two methods of coding—*references* to being better/more attractive to men or the current man in the consumers life and *phraseology* that stated, with words, the consumer would feel better about herself for using the product) in breast enhancement advertisements in *Cosmopolitan* magazine in the years 1990-2000. The results fascinated me. I further began to question how this image of breasts is accepted socially, why women aspired to obtain it (eighteen billion dollars in capital annually as of 2002), and the manner in which this 'ideal body/breast type' is marketed.

I spoke to my graduate studies academic advisor in the spring of 2002 while taking a Sociology class she taught. I explained to her my primary interest and she directed me to a number of readings and literature reviews. This was the beginning of writing this book.

Advertising to Women: 1890-1940

In researching this chapter, I read authors such as Naomi Wolf (The Beauty Myth), Stuart Ewen (Captains of Consciousness), Juliet Schor (The Overspent American), George Ritzer (Expressing America), and selected parts of books and articles written by Roland Marchand, Betty Friedan, and Jennifer Scanlon. I also began researching what has been published on the broad topic of advertising to women and I have primarily found research on: body image satisfaction questionnaires/focus groups, adolescent self-esteem, gender, and media influence, and finally advertising influencing eating disorders, low self-esteem, and drive to physical augmentation.

In this chapter, I explore the beginning of advertising to women and how it functioned through the first part of the twentieth century to lay a foundation for the ideal body type and 'beauty myth' of today.

Changing Physical Images of Women in the Media: 1940-1980

This chapter traces the shifts in beauty culture that occurred between 1940-1990. The 'ideal female beauty' presented by the media changed from being voluptuous and shapely to angular and thin. Content analysis studies are presented where the physique averages of models presented in popular women's magazines, *Playboy*, and the Miss America Pageant are compared to the 'average' women reported by the Society of Actuaries. Further studies demonstrate that women receive more images than men in advertising to stay in shape and thin. Finally, the chapter centers around the dramatic beauty image shift that occurred in the late 1960's when Twiggy, the tall and thin fashion model, completely changed the ideal female body type by taking the fashion world by storm.

How Do Biological Predispositions Influence Women to Undergo Cosmetic Surgery?

This chapter argues that women undergo 'beautification' surgeries and procedures in order to obtain valued resources in our society—primarily access to money, men, and jobs (jobs and money is what women have been historically denied). Our culture has set up a system that rewards certain physical traits of women and classifies others as deviant. Women are primarily judged by their appearance; therefore, I state that women conform to the 'standards' in order gain resources that society has deemed as 'rewards'. I further explore how biology has influenced this social competition.

I present the 'hypodermic model' of advertising given by the Critical Theory/ Frankfurt School. I wish to use this in presenting a view that consumers are passive and advertising agencies/corporations manipulate them in order to purchase products. Examples of authors who present this theory are Friedan (1963), Bordo (1993), and Ewen (1976, 1988). I also present the active consumer theory, which asserts that women are active, informed, and they have conscious and rational reasons for adopting the body discipline habits and changes that they do (Fiske 1989; Radway 1984; Campbell 1991; Rose 1990).

What is the 'Perfect' Female Physique and Who is Defining It?

This chapter is focused on the construction of social problems. Having already demonstrated how the concept of beauty changes throughout time in our culture, I wrote this chapter on what is defined as 'beautiful' for women in regards to physical shape. I use content analysis studies conducted on *Ladies Home Journal* and *Vogue* magazines, which yielded measurement data of the women models pictured.

What Institutions Have Emerged to Combat the Obesity Plague and Provide Products for Aesthetic Enhancement?

In this chapter, I explore what institutions have emerged in order to combat the 'fat plague' and provide products for physical enhancement. Media is the primary mode of passing along information and 'claims', so I used popular websites, magazines, and newspapers to understand what claims are being made by whom. I argue that the collectivity of the claims in advertising creates the 'fat plague' and other physical deviance first by marketing products that are a response to the problem; essentially, the problem is created after a solution has been proposed.

Frequency and Coding of Breast Enhancement Advertisements in *Cosmopolitan* and *Seventeen* Magazines: 1990-2000

In this chapter, I explore the way in which the media conveys the definition of success to women through advertising. Women are assimilated, through the media, to conform to the beauty image in order to secure a financially successful male partner; this is the definition of success. This is achieved by advertising to make women feel bad [self-esteem] or guilty about not having a certain product, thus defining the product as the vehicle to success. Further, I explore how advertising agencies target adolescent girls and women in different ways by conducting content analysis studies of Cosmopolitan and Seventeen magazines.

The Marijuana Tax Act

This is a bonus chapter not relating to anything else in the book. This chapter explores how the interests of a few powerful individuals at both the government and public level worked together to pass the Marijuana Tax Act of 1937. The propaganda campaign launched in the early 1930's that led to the passage of the Marijuana Tax Act permanently changed the way the public viewed the cannabis plant and marijuana smoking by rallying the emotions of the public against such substances. Further, this chapter explains the social standards of the time and the historical occurrences that led up to the Marijuana Tax Act being passed into law.

Advertising to Women: 1890-1940

For the past century, women's magazines have been one of the most powerful agents in both determining and changing women's roles. They have constantly glamorized (and consequentially defined) whatever the economy needed from women at the time—war movement, political agendas, and marketing demands (Wolf 1991:64). Throughout the past century, advertising agencies have been the puppeteer and women the marionette; the same agencies which have an agenda influenced by politics and the economy. Marketing agencies have historically used ads to reach consumers, but have specifically constructed ads to women on a calculated agenda—tugging on every emotion from self-esteem to sexuality acceptance—in order to make a profit.

Advertising to women in magazines reflected and influenced women's advances, as well as the idea of "the beauty myth" (a term coined by Naomi Wolf). Girton, Newnham, Vassar, Radcliffe, and many other institutions of higher education for women were founded in the 1860's. Historian Peter Gay wrote (in response to the opening of the higher education institutions), "Women's emancipation is out of control" (Wolf 1991: 62). At the same time, *The Queen* and *Harper's Bazaar* were established while the *English Women's Domestic Magazine* doubled to 50,000 in circulation. "The rise in women's magazines was brought about by large investments of capital combined with increased literacy and purchasing power of lower-middle—and working-class women" (Wolf 1991:62).

Magazines first accepted product advertisements from companies at the turn of the century; this was the very beginning of advertising to women and companies realizing that women had purchasing power in the economy. Magazines (both articles and advertisements), at that time, placed women in almost complete domestic bondage. Women actively participated in the war effort during World War I; when the war ended, both the soldiers and "the magazines returned to the home" (Wolf 1991:62). Women began spending more and were recog-

1

nized for making a majority of the consumption choices of the household because most women stayed home fulfilling the "traditional" role.

Advertising agencies began their hegemonic foothold in the magazine industry during the middle of World War I. They paid large amounts of money to advertise in leading magazines. In 1917, advertising agencies handled ninety-five percent of national advertising being promoted in magazines. By 1919, two-thirds of the revenue of magazines came from advertising agencies. "Due to its financial importance alone, then, advertising would secure a more influential role in the magazine's policy making…" (Scanlon 1995:172). This agreement was symbiotic in that advertisers could reach their targeted audience via the magazine median, and the magazine company received revenue from the agencies, which allowed them to keep their subscription rates low. Cyprus H. K. Curtis, the publisher of the *Ladies' Home Journal* in the early 1900's, once confided to an audience of manufacturers

> "Do you know why we publish the *Ladies' Home Journal?* The editor thinks it is for the benefit of American women. That is an illusion, but a very proper one for him to have. But I will tell you: the real reason, the publisher's reason, is to give you people who manufacture things that American women want and buy, a chance to tell them about your products" (Fowles 1996:37).

Advertisers recognized in the 1920's that women accounted for at least eighty percent of all consumer purchases. This is contradictory, demographically, in that women constituted a very small part of the nation's population, mass, and class segments. Advertising agencies constantly referred to women as "purchasing agents" of their families. This analogy suggests that women had the near complete responsibility for familial expenditures (Marchand 1985:66). Realizing that women were a major part of the consumer market, advertisers constantly kept the woman in the "limelight" in order to retain her business.

> "Although stereotyped characters abounded in the tableaux, the portrait of the American woman that emerged from the ads of the 1920's and 1930's is striking in its complexity. No other figure in the tableaux shifted roles and appearances so frequently. Yet the ultimate boundaries on the leading lady's scope of action were so clearly drawn that this apparent diversity of roles eventually came to seem less impressive" (Marchand 1985:167).

The previous century had defined the separation between work (men) and home; so much, in fact, that women had been polarized. The advertisements of the 1920's and 1930's only served to legitimize and facilitate this polarization. Men's proper sphere had been defined as work away from home. Work was a world of ambition, struggle, power, competition, and capitalism. The proper sphere of a woman, on the other hand, *was the home*. The work of the home was of caring and sentiment; a sanctuary for the husband to come home to. The "real world" and the "work of man" proceeded outside while the home was a "buffer against the harsher thrusts and shocks of progress" (Marchand 1985: 167-68).

Advertising agencies observed two phenomena: a woman's place (socially defined) was in the home, and women accounted for at least eighty percent of all consumer purchases. The agencies had to combine the two in regards to advertising to capture and hold the interest of the feminine market. In order to do this, the agencies developed the idea of "The Little Woman, G.P.A." (Marchand 1985:168-69). G.P.A was an acronym for 'General Purchasing Agent' and the motive was to praise women for their ability to save time and money for their family as holding the role. "As purchasing agents, women could command respect for exhibiting qualities previously honored primarily in men—capacities for planning, efficiency, and expert decision making" (Marchand 1985:168). N.W. Ayer and Son produced an ad that best represents (and pioneered) the idea. The ad places a woman at a 'domestic communications center', which is shown somewhat like a strategic planning room (similar to what we seen on CNN or movies when military officers are in the 'war room' with maps, charts, graphs, and books). The rest of the ad dignifies and legitimizes the job of a housewife by praising her for frugal and efficient decisions. Other ads, at that time, "disclosed the housewife planning expenditures or paying bills at her home desk and labeled her role 'manager' or 'executive'" (Marchand 1985:169).

Observing the success of the General Purchasing Agent campaign, advertisers turned to making advertising personal by attaching emotional and liberating qualities to personal items of women. Marketing reports of that time described how to manipulate housewives into becoming insecure consumers about household products. The focus was to stress guilt and therapeutic value of goods while simultaneously turning the mental association of housework into knowledge and skill (instead of 'brawn work'). The report concluded that commodities with "added psychological value" have no price limit (Wolf 1991:65). Thus, "specialized" cosmetics and other similar products began to flood the market.

The General Purchasing Agent model became a cornerstone of advertising to women because it not only dignified the role that so many women had been living (or arguably trapped in) for such a long time, but it praised them for their decision making process independent of the constant supervision of man (or her husband). For example, Piggy Wiggly stores congratulated women for their self-reliant skills in shopping. "For the women of today it is both easy and pleasant. Her new, wide knowledge of values, her new ability to decide for herself, is one of the wonders of the world we live in." By selecting products off the shelf with "no clerk to persuade her," proclaimed Piggy Wiggly, "she has astonished her husband...and the world." (Marchand 1985:169). It is amazing how advertisers designed the idea of "The Little Women, G.P.A.", but then reference her new-found (in the eyes of advertisement) accomplishment as astonishing her husband and the world, as if the thought of women having the brain-power to conduct such business never existed prior to the advertising proclamations. Even though the woman had found new independence through advertising imaging, she still was ultimately subordinate to and seeking the approval of the man of the household (and the male dominated society).

During this period of advertising to women, we begin to see a reoccurring theme of the success of a woman being dependent on the acceptance and approval of others. Marketing agencies used this idea to sell products to women by demonstrating that the outcome *from consuming or utilizing* the commodity would result in approval. Women's social roles were continually defined in terms of consumption. This subverted women to the whim of the advertisements because agencies told women, through their medium of advertising, what was available and what women *should* buy. "From the field of social psychology, advertising had borrowed the notion of the *social self* as a prime weapon in its arsenal. Here people defined themselves in terms set by the approval or disapproval of others" (McEwen 1976:179). In the Piggy Wiggly example, the woman 'astonished her husband and the world'. Later in this paper, we will learn how the social approval of others (primarily men) was used to sell products by creating a feeling of inadequacy and low self-esteem on a mass scale that had not existed before.

The truly efficient home manager's goal was to save both time and money. "A 'clever manager' not only claimed respect for her businesslike modernity, she also emancipated herself from withering isolation and cultural deprivation by creating time for outside activities" (Marchand 1985:70). This was accomplished by the push for women to turn household work into a science. Advertising then turned to emphasizing that women created more leisure time for themselves by effective management of household chores. With the innovation of technologies that were advertised to save time and thus create leisure time, women were left to explore how they would spend the newly found time.

As advertisements shifted to the new focus of demonstrating leisure time through innovative technologies and slightly away from the traditional 'managerial role', the advertised duties of the wife became interconnected with sex. One perfume ad stated that a woman's first duty is to attract men and "it does not matter how clever or independent you may be, if you fail to influence the men you meet, consciously or unconsciously, you are not fulfilling your fundamental duty as a woman…" (McEwen 1976:182). The advertising industry was placing great emphasis on sexual skills through the medium of consumption. McEwen concludes by stating, "If consumption management was a *role* of work, sexuality was, for women, a *duty* of leisure. The two, work and leisure, could not be separated. Consumption provided an idiom for the unity of the two" (McEwen 1976:182-83). Sex was considered a duty (of leisure) now that women had more leisure time thanks to innovative technologies. This idea of the woman needing to be a seductress set the later stage for development of women's sexuality through advertising.

Many new ads *showed* housewives enjoying their leisure time. This was accomplished by the product not present in the ad or subordinated by the woman. The focus was to make the product desirable by showing its ability to create leisure time for the woman, which she was enjoying as the centerpiece of the advertisement. The next question for marketing agencies was what women *wanted* to do with their leisure time, or what could be depicted in the ads. Companies would not want to show a women working in basement if she really wanted to be shopping—this could be suicide for a product. Women had been employed in advertising for quite some time, but were never (obviously) truly represented in equal numbers. In fact, "the 'main reason' that women were employed in advertising, Ruth Waldo of J. Walter Thompson acknowledged, was because they had 'intimate knowledge of women's habits and desires'" (Marchand 1985:34). By hiring women in advertising firms, the companies could find out what women wanted to do with their leisure time and they had women conducting the research as well as writing the ads.

The best way of understanding what women wanted to do with their leisure time, according to the advertising companies, is to look at the advertisements selling leisure time activities during the 1920's. Marchand studied the advertising campaign of the American Laundry Machine Corporation. The ads usually contained three or more illustrated testimonials of what women were choosing to pursue with their leisure time. From such content analysis, Marchand states, "Since the ads carry a large number of examples, we may be able to infer from them not only which activities women most desired, but also the boundaries of such desires. What these ads did *not* include may be as significant as what they specifically portrayed" (Marchand 1985:172).

Marchand found that leisure time devoted to reading and spending time with children outranked the other chosen activities of club activities (second), golf, sewing, part-time work outside of the home (third). No testimonial mentioned a career. A similar study between 1926 and 1928 reveals a heavier emphasis on spending time with and fostering companionship with one's children. A new expansion in advertising emerged, one to cultivating a feeling of companionship between mother and child. Ads showed women in warm scenes with their children off at picnics with them or romping through a field of wildflowers together (for examples). Marchand realizes that the leisure activities depicted may not have been representative of what women of that time chose to do, "nor will they reveal whether these choices for leisure time were authentic reflections of women's real attitudes" (Marchand 1985:172).

Tableaux characterized leisurely pursuits as forms of self-expression. More common were tableaux that brought women back full-circle to their traditional roles that demonstrated activities that made them better wives and mothers. Ads began to warn that the husband may outgrow the wife in "sophistication, class standing, and breadth of tastes and experiences" (Marchand 1985:175) in the highly bureaucratized business world that existed at the time. It was the responsibility of the women to remain stimulating social and intellectual companions. "They needed to preserve their youth so that they could beautify their husband's lives and keep pace with them during evenings of dancing and theater" (Marchand 1985:175). After this new advertisement push, women were not only to be business efficient (Little Woman, G.P.A.) in the home, but also must apply the time saved through modern management and technology to broadening her social interests, intellectual interests, and keep a youthful yet modern look.

We begin to observe another shift of advertising to women by studying the ads of the 1920's (prior to the bombardment of ads with women looking in mirrors). Carl Naether published popular studies on how to advertise to women in the 1920's. He discussed making women self-conscious about their bodies and how to direct this self-consciousness towards consumption. For example, he used an ad showing a woman fondling a breast-length strand of pearls. He stated that, "They [the pearls] center attention on those parts of the feminine body which they encircle and touch…[the ad] ingeniously compares women with these precious adornments, attributing to the former the qualities possessed by the latter" (McEwen 1976:180). Naether's studies directed women to be self-conscious of their sexuality in regards to both their husband and larger society:

"In the middle of her mechanically engineered kitchen, the modern housewife was expected to be overcome with issue of whether her "self", her "body", her personality were viable in the socio-sexual market that defined her job. Advertisements used pictures of veiled nudes and women in auto-erotic stances to encourage self-comparison and to remind women of the primacy of their sexuality" (McEwen 1976:179).

This concept was a pivotal point in advertising. Women were being encouraged to define themselves and further compete among themselves within the context of the ads marketed at that time. This was a completely new concept that set the stage for advertising to women through current times. Wolf illustrates what was *really* being plotted by marketing agencies by paraphrasing Friedan:

"...why is it never said that the really crucial function that women serve as aspiring beauties is *to buy more things for the body?* Somehow, somewhere, someone must have figured out that they will buy more things if they are kept in the self-hating, ever-failing, hungry, and sexually insecure state of being aspiring 'beauties'" (Wolf 1991:66).

"It was a world, in Roland Barthes's phrase, 'entirely constituted by the gaze of man', one in which 'man is everywhere around, he presses on all sides, he makes everything exist'. Lady Esther Face Cream expressed the idea more hauntingly: 'Men's eyes are magnifying mirrors'" (Marchand 1985:175). Advertisements showed women surrounded by mirrors, looking in mirrors, or being reflected in the mirror. This was a strategy used to create a notion of self-consciousness that had not existed on such a grand scale in advertising to woman previously. The mirror reminded each woman of the "central duty" of being beautiful, and that she was always under scrutiny not only by men, but now by herself as well (Marchand 1985:176).

McEwen agrees with Marchand, but furthers the ideal by adding that women could ensure fidelity and social (which could arguable by linked to professional) success by appearance, even more so than by their organizational ability. "...For women the imperative of beauty was directly linked to the question of job security-their *survival*, in fact, depended upon their ability to keep a husband, ads continually reminded women..." (McEwen 1976:178). Ads perpetuated this dynamic to women, as Marchand explains in the previous paragraph.

This is the emergence of yet another pivotal point in women's advertising—the ideal of being under constant scrutiny of a "man's gaze" and that a woman's central duty was to remain beautiful and youthful (all for her man).

Advertising artists had to create an idea of beauty for women to follow; products spoke of how a certain cream could invigorate the skin or how perfumes could make a woman smell more attractive, but a central idea of the beauty image had to be created for women to aspire to. The image created showed women of high-class and social desire to be

> "...slender, youthful, and sophisticated. Her finely etched facial features formed a slightly aloof smile, suggesting demure self-confidence in her obvious social prestige and her understated sexual allure. Attired elegantly, but not exotically, she stood tall and angular, her fingers and toes tapering to sharp points. In her role as a model of the proper feminine look, she gained credit for attracting the attention of women as much as men" (Marchand 1985:181).

Women of high fashion (and of high social status) appeared in advertisements as physically distinct from woman of lower social class and position. A central ideal of the ads was to show the women as having the characteristics to possess "conspicuous leisure" time". This is a theory by Thorstein Veblen meaning that one has the time to pursue interests in a non-productive function of time due to being wealthy enough to possess large amounts of leisure time. The overall appearance was grotesque and demented—very few women of that time resembled the women in the ads. "Fashion economist Paul Nystrom estimated in 1928 that only 17 percent of all American women were both 'slender' and over 5 feet 3 inches in height" (Marchand 1985:184).

Larger societal problems were born out of this method of advertising. Paul Nystrom estimated that not even a quarter of the female population 'fit' within the beauty myth constraints defined by advertising in 1928, yet women still judge themselves by this standard. This can only lead to body-image problems when attempting to emulate the women in the ads by purchasing the products. Wilson Brian Key, author of Media Sexploitation, sums up the issue the best by stating

> "Consider the American women's self-image in relation to her bodily endowments—biologically derived proportions over which most individuals have little power to change or modify. Young women with small breasts, for example, are quite likely to perceive themselves as deficient in personal value. American media establish and sustain the cultural models of desirable human configurations; women with heavy legs in America are also programmed automatically for a lifelong inferiority complex, as are generally larger, heavier, women" (Key 1976:36).

Advertising then began to correlate modernity with social and political freedom. "Expansive rhetoric that heralded women's march toward freedom and equality often concluded by proclaiming their victory only in the narrower realm of consumer freedom" (Marchand 1985:186). This was done by portraying educated and civil-minded women in advertisements and asking them, "What type of toothpaste do you vote for?" This was obviously a play on the then-recent decision concerning women's suffrage. An innovative new way of advertising to women emerged from this manner of equating consuming with freedom. It was pioneered by Edward L. Bernays, who believed that the best way to sell something was to pretend to sell something else. To demonstrate this idea, Bernays conducted a social experiment. He carefully selected ten women, put cigarettes in their hands, and sent them down Fifth Avenue in New York City on Easter Sunday, 1929. Bernays gave the women specific instructions on how and when to light the cigarette. He enlisted spokeswomen to describe the protest as an advance for feminism and labeled the incident "Torches of Freedom". He hired a photographer to take pictures. Bernays contrived this experiment so perfect that the incident made headlines across the country the following day and prompted heated debate about whether women should be allowed to smoke as freely as men did. He successfully changed the social context of cigarettes for history. Bernays hid one secret throughout his plan—he worked for the American Tobacco Company and was using the "march" as a way to expand the tobacco market to women. Bernays successfully equated social freedom and liberation for women with smoking cigarettes; he sold women something (cigarettes) by pretending it was something else (freedom) (Gladwell 1998:66-67).

Despite advances politically in women's rights and the marketing agencies attempts to liberate women through consumer spending, women still did not escape the responsibility of the "home". Equating political and social freedom to choosing toothpaste (or smoking) only served to further the subordination of women at the home and ultimately held them responsible for familial matters. Advertising, through the 1920's and 30's, reminded women that they were not only responsible for making thrifty decisions with the household budget, but were also required to create leisure time through smart purchasing that would allow them to spend time perfecting skills to keep their husband intellectually and culturally stimulated. Not only that, but women were also constantly under the scrutiny of themselves (by the mirror) as well as by men and that they should never "let him down" or allow him to loose interest. Responsibility for social, marriage, and familial management became the sole responsibility of the woman through advertising.

The claim of women's roles had come full circle in the tableaux. The efficient home manager, G.P.A. was first, then the personal modernity afforded by leisure time, followed by fashion modernism and the ideal beauty type, and finally back to the cornerstone of the house and the backbone of the marriage and family.

Where did advertising to women go after the original pioneering of capturing the female audience, and what did this mean for stereotyped image of women sold by the media? I plan to cover advertising to women from 1940 to present times in my next paper, but I would like to give you a few examples of later changes. Women's activist groups became very angry at the way in which women were portrayed in the media. They argued that "many pressures conspire to deny women the variety of life patterns open to men" (Sexton and Haberman 1974:41). Stereotypes were defined as "the happy and diligent housewife who strives for whiter wash and shinier floors; the beautiful but dependent social companion, and the girl who wished to be blonde, thin, or have a characteristic she does not naturally possess" (Sexton and Haberman 1974:41). Based on these dimensions, Sexton and Haberman conducted a longitudinal (twenty years) content analysis research project based on 1,827 advertisements from the magazines Good Housekeeping, Look, Newsweek, Sports Illustrated, and TV Guide. They concluded that the overall results appeared to corroborate the feminist activist group charges that the role of women reflected in advertisements was very narrow. Sexton and Haberman concluded that women being alluring, decorative, or traditional was still an essential element to sell products. There was a slight increase in the role of women working, but the tasks still remained "traditional". There was, however, a substantial decrease in ads portraying women as a housewife or a mother (Sexton and Haberman 1974).

Another study of content analysis coding for 729 ads from eight magazines from the publishing week of April 18, 1970 revealed similar findings. Women were rarely shown in working roles—this was ironic since, at that time, women comprised thirty-three percent of the full-time work force but only twelve percent of ads portrayed women in working roles. If they did work, they were shown in "traditional" roles such as a stewardess or schoolteacher. Women rarely ventured far from the house by themselves or with other women in the advertisements as well, but they did smoke, drink, and travel (primarily in the company of the man) (Courtney and Lockeretz 1971).

These two selected studies revealed that the advancement of portraying women in realistic roles progressed slowly from 1940 to 1970. Women were still portrayed as the submissive sex and as decorative objects; this portrayal was a base for selling products. Yet further, from 1959 to 1989 women were featured decreasingly as homemakers, increasingly without a male present, and increasingly in a decorative pose (Knowles 1996:211). The main shift of advertising to women from the 1940's to the modern day was getting women out of domicile and submissive (to men) roles and portraying them as decorative and sexual objects. The conception of 'beauty' changes numerous times during this time. In the next chapter, we will discover how the media demonstrated the idea of 'beauty' from 1940-1989 in various media sources.

Changing Physical Images of
Women in the Media:
1940-1980

"One hypothesis that is common to a number of these mechanisms is that in the late 20th century American women are under pressure to be unrealistically thin" (Silverstein et. al. 1986:520).

"For example, 'perfect' breast size and hip size oscillates with the current trend in the fashion world" (Mazur 1986:281-303).

"At the current time it is not possible to prove that the media actually cause women to be obsessed and dissatisfied with their bodies or to calculate the relative importance of the media in this process compared with other sources of messages to women, such as fathers, husbands, physicians, and friends" (Silverstein et. Al. 1986:531-532).

"Thus, advertising is socially necessary as the underwriter of both information and entertainment in mass communication" (Walker quoted in Sinclair 1987:67).

Throughout the twentieth century, we can observe many changes in the world of the fashion and beauty industry that is primarily marketed to women. In particular, the physical shape and characteristics of the women portrayed in advertisements have changed. In an earlier paper that I wrote, I presented how women were portrayed in fashion advertisements from 1890 to 1940. In this paper, I plan to explore how women are portrayed in the media from 1940 to modern times (research primarily ending in 1980). The female image in the media has changed from being voluptuous and curvaceous in the 1940's and 1950's to being busty and narrow-hipped from the late 1960's through the 1980's. Specific examples of women have been used as embodying the media representation of the body type presented at a given time, and they conversely are illustrative of a change by being compared to the later portrayed image. I will present studies that have measured physical traits of media samples of women over a definitive time and then compared the findings to both measurements of real women over the same time period *and* media images of women of previous decades. Finally, I will present how the changing image has correlated with the preferred body size of women by comparing two subsequent generations of women.

It is sometimes claimed by advertising agencies that the media only give people what they want. If this were true, then the individuals that make decisions concerning what women want from the media believe that many women desire the given presentations. Furthermore, such presentations would only feed back to affect other women.

> "Thus, present-day women who look at the major mass media are exposed to a standard of bodily attractiveness that is slimmer than that presented for men and that is less curvaceous than that presented for women since the 1930's. This standard may not be promoted only in the media and it may not even originate in the media, but given the popularity of television, movies, and magazines…the media are likely to be among the most influential promoters of thin standards" (Silverstein et. al. 1986:531).

Bergerson and Senn (1998) state that socio-cultural norms have played a large part in the manifestation and the propagation of negative body image. Women are taught that appearance is the most important part of their lives, it is more important than what they think, and that appearance affects social opportunities. "Women get the message early that they must look good in order…to please men" (Bergerson and Senn 1998:386).

The obsession of North American women with diet and thinness took hold in the 1920's (Marchand 1985, Wolf 1991). "Having the appropriately sized and proportioned body increased a woman's opportunities for value and esteem from herself, her female peers, males, and society" (Torrens 1998:29). To attain success in society in these dimensions, a woman must have control over her body. Being able to shape it to fit the ideal body type of the given time will result in personal and professional fulfillment; the right job, mate, and home will accrue if she has the proper look (Torrens 1998).

Thinness is strongly related to social class in advertisements. Women in advertisements that fit the given ideal type body throughout the twentieth century have been portrayed as financially successful (Marchand 1985). Often times the ads are promoting an image that links social, financial, and emotional success with a product that, in some manner, gives control of how the body looks to the consumer of that product (Bordo 1993). Rarely do we see wealthy and financially successful women in advertisements presented as overweight or 'out of control' of their bodies. Just as image has been theorized (Bergerson and Senn 1998, Torrens, 1998) to affect social opportunities, being thin is related to social class. "Furthermore, for North American women, higher social class is strongly related to thinness and dieting" (Garner et. al. 1980:483).

After the end of World War I, hems were raised and waistlines lowered (Laver 1963). According to Lamb et. al., dresses of the 1920's have few curves and the ideal figure for a woman was boyish and flat-chested ('flapper' model). The 1930's glamorized women such as Mae West and Jean Harlow (both curvaceous). During the 1940's, the ideal type was that of a 'sweater girl', such as Lana Turner or Jayne Russell (becoming more curvaceous towards the end of the decade). In the 1950's and 1960's, Marilyn Monroe (curvy as they get as a size 12 with measurements of 35-22-35) was the popular type with the 'svelte' figures of Audrey Hepburn and Grace Kelly becoming the ideal in the late part of the decade and carrying through the mid 1960's. "'Twiggy', in 1966 became the fashion sensation and a new ideal. With her increasing popularity, the voluptuous figure idolized in the past seemed to lose its desirability" (Lamb et. al. 1993:347).

Mellican (1995) adds that there has been pressure on women throughout history to conform to prevailing fashions and standards of beauty. He confers that there have been 'rapid shifts' from the Lillian Russell/Marilyn Monroe standard, which was voluptuous and curvaceous, to the 1920's Flapper/1960's Twiggy standard, which was unisex slim, to today's mix of full breasted yet narrow-hipped woman. "The era of the cinch belt, the pushup bra, and Marilyn Monroe could be viewed, for the body, as an era of 'resurgent Victorianism'. It was also the last coercively normalizing body-ideal to reign before boyish slenderness began its ascendancy in the mid-1960's" (Bordo 1993:208). The one constant in these shifting ideals is that they present a standard that is very difficult, if not impossible, for most women to achieve. McKinely and Hyde believe that women "internalize cultural body standards so that the standards appear to originate from the self and believe that achieving these standards is possible even in the face of considerable evidence to the contrary" (McKinley and Hyde 1996:183).

This change from the 1940s to the 1990s did not occur overnight. If we look at a few of the studies conducted during this time in regards to the changing body image of women in the media, we see that the change was gradual and progressive until 'Twiggy' erupted on the fashion scene in the late 1960's (31-22-32 measurements and barely ninety pounds on her 5' 6" frame). With her lack of curves that characterized the earlier, popular female media representations, a new ideal body type was born. This created a profound change that redefined the ideal female body image in the media for the years to come, and eventually became the image to be expected by consumers.

In our country, we have seen a successful advertising campaign of the ideal thinness by the fashion industry. This body type (almost anorexic) is not an isolated phenomenon, but instead has become the idealized standard of beauty and fashion since the 1970's. "Today, the average fashion model—our representative of the ideal type—weighs 23 percent less than the average American woman" (Torrens quoting Wolf 1991:184).

Several ten year-old boys were shown photos of some fashion models on the magazine show "20/20". The models were thin, but the poses they were in were such that a small bulge of hip was sticking out or flesh was mildly bulging due to the posturing. The boys pointed to the 'bulges' and hips and pronounced the models 'fat'. Susan Bordo, upon watching this series of events, comments

> "Watching the show, I was appalled at the boys' reaction. Yet I could not deny that I had also been surprised at my own current perceptions while re-viewing female bodies in movies from the 1970's; what once appeared slender and fit now seemed to be loose and flabby. *Weight* was not the key element in these changed perceptions—my standards had not come to favor thinner bodies—rather, I had come to expect a tighter, smoother, more contained body profile" (Bordo 1993:187-188).

Some advertisements portray women in very traditional roles. I thought that the women's movement of the 1960's would influence the occupation and independent status of women in advertisements for the following years, but I found the contrary to be true. Courtney and Lockeretz (1971) studied 729 ads from the week of April 18, 1970 in the magazines *Life, Look, Newsweek, New Yorker, Saturday Review, Time, US News and World Report*, and the April edition of *Reader's Digest*. Using content analysis, they found that the advertisements rarely showed women in working roles. At that time, thirty-three percent of full-time workers were women whereas only twelve percent of the women in the advertisements were working. Women were shown in traditional roles and, when employed in the ads, were shown as primarily clerks and stewardesses. Fifty-eight percent were shown as 'entertainers'—women in decorative or familial roles. The ads further portrayed women as rarely venturing far from home by themselves or with other women; although they do smoke, drink, and travel, it is primarily in the company of men.

I feel that the best way to present how the media representation of the female body has changed is to look at longitudinal content analysis studies. Through production of quantitative data, we can learn how the change has occurred. In conducting these studies, a few of the research teams also observed that advertisements for dieting and food products far outnumbered promotions in women's magazines than in men's. These data will be presented as well.

Torrens states that, "Weight loss advertising is an enormous industry that supports an even more enormous set of commercial enterprises aimed at focusing women's attention and energies on their bodies" (Torrens 1998:27). In the early years (1920-1945), women were believed to make up as much as eighty percent of all consumer purchases (Marchand 1985), and advertisers quickly constructed a market directed at women. Marchand states that in the eyes of advertisers that the characteristic consumer demonstrated such qualities as "capriciousness, irrationality, passivity, and conformism" (Marchand 1985:69). Emotions as the "lowest common human denominator" were received as the most appropriate avenue of persuasion (Marchand 1985:69).

Silverstein et. al. (1986) conducted a study in order to demonstrate the following three things: 1.) That the current standard of attractiveness for women in the media is slimmer than for men 2.) That the standard now is slimmer than it has been in the past, and 3.) That these findings apply to major media. They conducted content analysis studies of leading women's magazines to demonstrate this—*Family Circle, Ladies Home Journal, Redbook,* and *Woman's Day.* They used the same research design in four leading men's magazines—*Field and Stream, Playboy, Popular Mechanics,* and *Sports Illustrated.*

In order to demonstrate that a slim standard of bodily attractiveness is perpetuated by the media, it is necessary to demonstrate three things:

1. That the media promote a slimmer, more weight-conscious standard for women than for men.

2. That the standard of bodily attractiveness for women is slimmer now than it has been in the past.

3. That points one and two apply to many examples of the media.

They concluded that, "the results of the content analysis provide strong support for the hypothesis that women receive more messages to be slim and stay in shape than do men" (Silverstein et. al. 1986:525). The advertisements for diet foods in the women's magazines far outnumbered those in the men's. They used forty-eight magazines (each for both men and women) and found that *sixty-three* ads appeared in women's compared to *one* in men's. The same is true for the 'body' category—articles dealing with shape or size and advertisements for non-food figure enhancing products—*ninety-six* in women's magazines and *eight* in men's. Women's magazines also advertised for food at a rate 100 times greater than for men's magazines (1,179 to 15).

Furthering their study, Silverstein et. al. measured the changes in the standards of bodily attractiveness over time for women. They state the following:

1. It is necessary to use material that has left a record since the turn of the century.

2. It is necessary to use material that can be considered to portray the types of bodies that women might use as a standard.

They used photographs from the magazines *Ladies Home Journal* and *Vogue*. After controlling for numerous sources of error that result from this method chosen, they ultimately used ratios between various parts of the bodies depicted in the photographs only of women in underwear or bathing suits—bust to waist and hips to waist. For both magazines, they began with the year 1901 and subsequently used issues every four years thereafter to end in 1981. From the findings, the researchers concluded that the magazines correlated in their depiction of women—.91 (p < .01). They found that the "curvaceous" look (higher ratios of difference between coded body parts) was prominent in the beginning of the century, but steadily decreased until a low hit in 1925. "By the late 1940's, the ratio had climbed back up, never coming close to the 1901 ratio, but increasing approximately one-third in both magazines. Beginning in 1949, the ratio dropped again, reaching the 1920's level in the late 1960's and the 1970's" (Silverstein et. al. 1986:528).

Garner et. al. (1980) conducted a study comparing the height, weight, bust, and hips of *Playbody* centerfolds, contestants of the Miss America pageant, and diet articles in six popular women's magazines over the past twenty years.

Playboy magazine allowed Garner et. al. to recover the height, weight, and body measurements of all 240 monthly playmates which appeared from 1959-1978. The average age, height, weight, bust, waist, and hip measurements are presented in the writing. "In addition, the average weight of the playmates was compared to population means reported by the 1959 Society of Actuaries" (Garner et. al. 1980:484). The yearly mean weight for the centerfolds was significantly less than the corresponding population mean. The changes within the playmates over the twenty-year time period is most important: "While absolute weight did not decline because heights were increasing, a regression analysis showed that the percent of average weight for age and height decreased significantly over the 20 yr [sic]. These absolute declines in measurements occurred in women who were increasing in height" (Garner et. al 1980:485). In 1968, the playmates had a weight lowest in regards to the population mean. We see, through this study, that the height of the playmate increased while her weight decreased along with the playmate weight being significantly lower than the women's mean population weight.

Height, weight, and age data were derived for both the winners and the contestants of the Miss America Pageant from 1959 through 1978. The means were calculated and, once again, compared to the means reported by the 1959 Society of Actuaries. Garner et. al. found that contestants declined yearly in weight by .28 pounds and the winners declined yearly in weight by .37 pounds. Average height in both winners and contestants drastically jumped (two inches) from 1968 to 1970, along with average waist size increasing two inches from 1960 to 1978.

Garner et. al. further analyzed the data and thought that maybe population norms had changed over the twenty-year period, so this may account for the decrease in weight. "Thus, the 1959 average weight statistics from the Society of the Actuaries were compared with the recent actuarial data from the Society (1979)" (Garner et. al. 1980:487). When comparing the data, they found an average weight increase of .3 pounds per year over the twenty-year period.

Garner et. al. then selected six popular women's magazines for the years of 1959 through 1978. The numbers of articles (not tabulations and promotions) about dieting and weight loss were calculated (mean) for each year. They found that the number doubled over the twenty-year time period with the largest jump being between 1968 (twenty-two articles) to 1970 (forty articles).

Garner et. al. concluded that, "these results strongly support the idea that there has been a gradual but definite evolution in the cultural body ideal shape for women over the past 20 years. Particularly within the past 10 years [1968-1978], there has been a shift in the ideal standard toward a thinner size" (Garner et. al. 1980:489). The Playboy data further demonstrate that measurements have moved to a more 'tubular' body form. The movement towards a thinner body shape in *Playboy* playmates and Miss America Pageant winners contrasts with the increase in weight of the female population norm given by the Society of the Actuaries. "Thus while the magazine centerfolds, Pageant participants, and presumably the prevailing female role models have been getting thinner, the average women of a similar age have become heavier" (Garner et. al. 1980:490). Lamb et.

al. agrees by stating, "It has been demonstrated that the women who embody the ideal of feminine beauty in the American culture (beauty queens and models) have become thinner over the last couple of decades to the point that the ideal figure is actually below the actuarial norm" (Lamb et. al. 1993:348).

Lamb et. al. (1993) administered questionnaires to a selected group of individuals over the age of thirty-nine, a group of people in a pre-retirement village, and to a group of college students representative of a geographic region in our nation (with most from southern, middle-class, Protestant backgrounds) [this is all the information about this demographic that the study provided]. Men and women were evenly represented in the sample. The older cohort was raised in the 1940's and 1950's (Marilyn Monroe and Susan Hayworth era). The younger cohort, in college, was raised directly after the "Twiggy" era; the thin, anorexic and tubular shape became popular in advertising (1980's). The questionnaire contained five body silhouettes (Stunkard Body Shape Figure Scale) that were shaped from excessively thin to overweight. The respondents were then asked questions and instructed to reply using the silhouette that correctly identified their perception. Men had male silhouettes and females had female silhouettes.

This model was chosen in order to compare the perceptions of the older cohort and younger cohort that were raised during times when the ideal female body type presented by the media was dramatically different. Lamb et. al. wanted to discover male perceptions of female body types (both wanted and realistic) and female perceptions of body types (both what men want and how they perceive themselves).

The results were that college women, older women, and older men considered their present body shape to be heavier than their ideal body figure. Only college men were satisfied, and actually reported wanting to be larger. Women believed men of their own cohort preferred very thin women, and the ideal figure reported by the men was not as thin as the ideal figure women reported wanting themselves. Older women reported that a more curvaceous and fuller figure is 'most attractive to the opposite sex', where the younger women picked a much thinner silhouette than the older women as being 'most attractive to the opposite sex". "Yet the cohort differences found in this study might reflect a true cohort effect exemplified in the Twiggy phenomenon of the middle to late 1960's" (Lamb et. al. 1993:355). For the older subjects, the desirability for a fuller body figure, such as the body type Marilyn Monroe (that was the prevailing beauty when they were growing up), would reflect this preference for a fuller figure and a different set of values by the older subjects compared to the stereotypes of desirable body figures of the younger cohort.

Spillman and Everington (1988) gave questionnaires to 234 university students in order to examine "the relation between certain behavioral characteristics and female body-build somatotypes…The purpose of the study was to investigate whether thin images presented by the media today are consistent with earlier body-image stereotypes or whether current stereotypes are different. That is, is this image now perceived by college students as possessing more desirability?" (Spillman and Everington 1989:887).

The respondents were given silhouettes representing three different female body types. The ectomorph build is thin, the endomorph build is fat, and the mesomorph build is somewhat muscular. They were then asked to assign each of the given twenty-four characteristics the three female builds (somatotypes).

The endomorph was regarded as the sloppiest dresser, under the most stress, and most likely to be depressed. It was also chosen to be the most likely to have a menial job and not be a professional, such as a lawyer or a dentist. The mesomorph type was attributed with the most positive characteristics, such as strength, health, happiness, friendship, and intelligence; however, it was also chosen for aggression. Contrary to previous findings, the ectomorphic body build was attributed with positive characteristics. This build was seen as most sexually appealing, having the most dates, exercising the most, and being the most knowledgeable about nutrition. This type was also associated with being the most concerned about appearance. When asked what type they would like to be, women chose the ectomorph and men chose the mesomorph, even though both sexes reported they see themselves as the mesomorph. Of note, there was no significant difference between men (44) and women (190) on any of the twenty-four questions addressing behavioral characteristics. Spillman and Everington concluded, "the findings support the notion that women college students are preoccupied with images of thinness and fitness" (Spillman and Everington 1989:889).

In conclusion, many studies have been presented that direct attention to what appears to be a trend. From the years of 1950 to 1980, we learn that the media image of a female weighed less, became taller, slimmed down in the hips, gained inches around the waist, yet remained busty. The main years that we observe this change, through analysis of quantitative data, are from the mid 1960's through the mid 1970's. We also see that ads for dieting products and food both drastically increase in women's magazines, especially from the late 1960's through the 1970's. We further learn that 'Twiggy', presented as angular in form with narrow hips, tall height, busty, and 'anorexic' in appearance, came to the fashion scene and became popular in the late 1960's. Researchers have studied college women to learn that they prefer a very thin body type and believe that men prefer this as well, yet perceive themselves as a heavier somatotype (mesomorph). When compared to the same study conducted on older women, we learn that they prefer a more full and curvaceous body and believe that men prefer the same. This disparity in preference and perceived desire of men could be attributed to the different ideal female body type presented by the media during different decades, as the quantitative data and research clearly demonstrates.

How Do Biological Predispositions Influence Women to Undergo Cosmetic Surgery?

"I came to see Dr. X for the holiday season. I have important business parties, and the man I'm trying to get to marry me is coming in from Paris" (Morgan 2000:153) [Quote in regards to why a woman chose have cosmetic surgery performed].

"[Now, women are being pressured to see plainness or being ugly as a form of pathology. Consequently, there is a strong pressure] to be beautiful in relation to the allegedly voluntary nature of 'electing' to undergo cosmetic surgery" (Morgan 2000:157).

If we look at the root of all conflict in nearly any situation, it can be traced to resources. The actors involved are trying to obtain or defend the resource that is valued by both conflicting parties. For example, we did not go to the Persian Gulf in the early 1990's to liberate Kuwait from the invasion of Sadaam Hussein. Kuwait is a geopolitical strategic location in the Middle East and has abundant natural resources of petroleum (Kemp 1998). The United States sent the Contras down to Nicaragua in Central America not as a means to thwart 'communism' from taking hold militarily, but rather as the Reagan administration viewing the Sandinistas as being too independent and not buckling under our economic interest of importing their rich mineral resources; the Pan-American Highway also passes through the country. (Robinson 1997).

My critique of the nature verses nurture (or the biological imperative verses culture) argument is that I find very few centrists in my literature reviews and class readings. The majority of authors take one side or the other. This thought process follows suit for the Creation verses Evolution argument, and if you have read any Ann Rice novel (Memnoch the Devil is most exemplary) you understand that she believes that both equally influenced each other. I propose that

22

biology coupled with culture form us as social beings. I do not believe that it is neither completely biology nor completely culture, but that we are born with biological predeterminations that influence our preferences and decisions socially.

Resources are anything that is valued by two interested parties, although one has more than the other. Liberals believe that a just society is one that allows individuals to maximize their self-fulfillment. Liberals further state that the 'right' must be given priority over the 'good' because, "…our whole system of individual rights is justified because these rights constitute a framework within which we can all choose our separate goods, provided we do not deprive others of theirs" (Tong 1998:11). It then becomes a challenge to create a society where everyone is fulfilling their wants and needs without depriving others of theirs. Valued resources are important to individuals. Tong states,

> "For if it is true, as most liberals claim, that resources are limited and each individual, even when restrained by altruism, has an interest in securing as many resources as possible, then it will be a challenge to create political, economic, and social institutions that maximize the individual's freedom without jeopardizing the community's welfare" (Tong 1998:11).

This theory is the base of what I am proposing in this paper. I argue that men, in a particular social status group in our culture, are valued resources for whom women who subscribe to the 'ruling culture ideology of beauty' *and* who have plastic surgery are competing.

I am focusing on plastic surgery because it has permanent effects, appeals to a specific audience, and is based in the knowledge that the participant subscribes to dominating patriarchal beauty myths by undergoing the procedure. The 'ruling culture ideal of beauty' is outlined in the previous papers presenting beauty presentations of women through media avenues. I use 'ruling' because these images are presented by the media who have the financial resources to promote the interests of those *with* the media resources. I do not believe that what is considered beauty in the media is a cultural Truth; rather, it is racially, age, and genetically biased. I argue that that subscribing to this ideology influences a woman's decision to have plastic surgery based on the 'inadequacy tactic' used to market and sell the beautifying product. In other words, if one believes that the media sets the standard for beauty, then the individual could feel inadequate and this could influence the decision to undergo plastic surgery.

Women are competitive and are aggressive. Biologically, I argue that any living entity in this world is competitive and aggressive because all are trying to survive while gathering the most resources that are required for it's survival. The requirements are often a skewed line between biology and society. For example, one may argue that Bill Gates does not need his empire and company monopoly to survive. This is true from a biological standpoint as he could subsist on a much smaller income (to meet the basic necessities of life), but his resources gain him respect, prestige, and honor in our society (and throughout other industrialized countries for that matter). Our society has a mode of production called capitalism, and the adage of 'he who dies with the most toys wins' holds true as a cultural value. We believe that money will buy us respect and prestige in the eyes of 'others'. Money can ensure that an individual and their family will always have what material items they need and want.

I am going to use media examples throughout this paper. This is because I believe that the media influences all of us in some way, and some more than others. If one subscribes to the media standard, then I feel it is appropriate to use the standard against itself. Nothing illustrates the resource argument more clearly than the new Fox reality television show, "Joe Millionaire" that aired in the Spring of 2003. Joe is a construction worker earning 19,000 dollars a year at the age of twenty-eight. He is posing as a man who recently inherited fifty million dollars and is looking for a wife. Fox put 'Joe' and twelve women in a chateau in France where the selection process begins. The question that Fox asks is, "Will Joe's final selection love him for the money or his personality?" Woman would not volunteer to go to France and compete with eleven others in hopes to marry if it were not for the money. I make this statement because all of the women are in their mid-twenties, attractive by societal standards, and are working professionals; I doubt they are short of available dating partners. This falls in line with the stereotypes of successful men marrying 'trophy wives'. We can see examples of this daily in the media. For instance, take Rod Stewart (with his second Victoria Secret model) or Anna Nicole Smith—she was awarded eighty-five million dollars of the estate of her late husband who was in his eighties when he died after they were only married for five months.

Diane Fossey, the chronicler of the central African mountain gorillas, had been studying a particular gorilla band for nine years when she noticed that one of the babies had disappeared. Acting on a hunch, she sifted through the excrement of the tribe that had been left for a few days. After following this group for nine years, Fossey and her assistants could identify which dung came from which gorilla. Finally, Fossey found 133 bone fragments from an infant gorilla in the dung of the dominant female and her eight-year-old daughter. Effie, the dominant female, committed this act right before she gave birth to her fourth baby. Killing the baby she did ensured that Effie would have the most children in the tribe; therefore, she asserted her position as dominant female and ensured her children's position in the ruling class. Effie acted like an ambitious wife in a harem who was eliminating the competition. Livia was one of the many wives of Augustus Caesar in Rome. She managed to eliminate the competition within the harem by tarnishing the reputation of the others and, at times, poisoning them to death. Rome was shifting power to a one-man emperorship at the time, and becoming the dominant female ensured that her children would inherit the power. Augutus had many children by other women, but Livia eliminated them through poisoning and hiring murderous help. What drove Effie and Livia was strictly maternal—the desire to give every advantage to her young (Bloom 1995:31-33). I argue that this same concept and maternal instinct can be brought into the resource argument. Women in our society want to be the "dominant female" in order to ensure the best chances of social survival for their children. Marrying rich will ensure this. Watching the women argue on the show "Joe Millionaire" demonstrates this as well. The women were manipulative towards each other and constantly trying to out rank the competition on a daily basis. Getting selected to marry a millionaire out of competition puts the woman in the same rank as Livia and Effie. Bloom further states,

> "Technically, this is called sexual selection. The female of a species develop a craving for a certain kind of guy, and all the males compete to live up to the female ideal. Lady peacocks adore hunks with towering blue tails, so peacock gentlemen sport foppish plumes. Lady bowerbirds swoon over bachelors with an architectural flare, so bowerbird males turn sticks and scraps into Taj Mahal" (Bloom 1995:33).

I understand that the argument "chicken or the egg first" is conjecture and unanswerable. Is it males responding to female selections or females responding to the males that give them the most adaptable offspring? Male penguins have an interesting way of attracting a mate during the 'season'. For male penguins, having the tallest stack of rocks is a way to guarantee that it will mate. The ground is frozen where penguins habitat and female penguins lay their eggs in a nest of rocks. The closer the nest is to the ground, the more chance the eggs have of freezing. Thus, male penguins build the rocky nest as high as they can and patiently await a female penguin to come by in search of a mate. What is more interesting is that the males congregate in one area and scamper to get rocks to build the tallest nest. The males try to knock down their neighbors rocks, attempt to steal them, and will occasionally get into altercations before the female penguins come to the known location of the male suitors. The male penguins are fighting over the resource of getting the most rocks to build the tallest nest in order to attract a mate. They defend it to the death. The penguins with the least amount of rocks or no nest at all do not mate and therefore do not pass on their genes to the next generation (Stokes and Dee Boersma 2000). They have lost the valued resource.

The male gray tree squirrel has a manipulative way of catching a mate. There is a bird that is a natural predator of the gray tree squirrel and makes a specific noise when it is about to attack. Since the bird has vision that is based on movement, the squirrel will freeze still until the perceived threat has vanished. The female gray tree squirrel is naturally faster than the male in running around and jumping from trees; this has evolved from running away from three to five suitors at any given mating time. The male squirrel that gets to mate with the female uses the natural predator's noise to his advantage. Some males have adapted a physical trait that allows them to reproduce the sound of the natural predator. That squirrel will make the noise and all the gray squirrels freeze. Then, the male reproducing the noise will continue to pursue the female and mate her; all the other males in pursuit have lost (Lishak 1982).

These actions follow in line with Charles Darwin's theory of natural selection where only the most adaptable survive. Somewhere along the line of biological evolution, female penguins figured out that the higher elevation of a nest correlated with a better chance of their young surviving. The females then 'selected' the mates who 'got it' and built tall nests. The male gray tree squirrel adapted to reproducing the sound of a natural predator and used this to advantage during the mating season. In both examples, the animals were competing over resources. The most adaptable figured out how to get or develop the resource despite competition.

I argue that Darwin's theory of natural selection can be applied to social contexts. We have biological impulses and have to find a socially acceptable means in which to both achieve our biological goals and survive in society. I argue that women get plastic surgery as a way to attract the best mate and acquire the best resources for themselves (and possibly their offspring) through socially acceptable means.

Our mode of production is capitalism. Everything we do in our culture has a base root in our mode of production. Capitalism is competition for and accumulation of resources. Often times human beings are seen as objects as we have a current quasi-religion of materialism where objects are our God (Christmas, or how about 'Black Friday' [problems with verbal discourse here?]). We relate to each other as we relate to the goods we buy; expendable and temporary. Competition fuels capitalism by creating 'new and improved' products that are sold to us as necessities for survival. We must constantly replace or upgrade, trash or eliminate. What is the end result of this constant competition? The results are financial resources and success of the company that the employee works for. Everything under capitalism is struggling and competing for survival and advancement, whether it is a social structure (company/organization) or an individual.

Despite the advancement of women's rights and the consciousness that has been raised about such issues since the 1960's, our culture still socializes women to marry and have children. Girls are saturated with this ideology from a very young age. Everything from Disney fairytales to 'girl' toys being dolls reinforces this value held by our culture. For instance, let's look at the popular Disney movie *Snow White*. The evil stepmother asks the mirror, "Who is fairest of them all?" In asking this, she is obviously competing for position and power. Morgan states that, "The affirmation of her beauty brings what is privileged heterosexual affiliation, privileged access to forms of power unavailable to the pain, the ugly, the aged, the barren" (Morgan 2000:153). As girls mature to adolescence, they become cognoscente of their bodies in relation to others their age and the media images that present a dominant white, European body-type as the only true beauty. When women reach full adulthood, they feel pressure from family members and friends to marry and start a family. When a man wants to marry a woman, he is supposed to ask her father for permission (cultural value). Her father then 'gives her away', and the wife changes her last name to her husband's. This is clearly transference of ownership, as if the woman is the property of men her whole life.

A woman's value as a social being is still only as strong as her husband's occupation. For example, a woman could be a lawyer yet people will say, "She is that lawyer married to a garbage man". Women are not taught to be autonomous or independent in our society. Our culture assigns values to men and women differently in a dichotomous approach. Tong discusses how Betty Friedan describes masculine and feminine traits in *The Second Stage* as

> "...culturally feminine so-called beta styles of thinking and acting, which emphasize "fluidity, flexibility and interpersonal sensitivity," and as culturally masculine so-called alpha styles of thinking and acting, which stress "hierarchal, authoritarian, strictly task-oriented leadership based on instrumental, technological rationality" (Tong 1998:29).

Men are independent, strong, assertive, and have fortitude. Women are caring, dependent, and nurturing. The values assigned to women are taught to be signs of weakness to men in our society, therefore setting up an exclusionary ideology of finding self-definition by what values men are 'not', and also which so happen to be seen as 'weakness'. "Mill...claimed that society's *ethical* double standard hurts women. Most of the "virtues" extolled in women are, in fact, negative character traits impeding women's progress toward personhood" (Tong 1998:18). Men are taught that these values are exclusively feminine (as defined culturally) and that 'men do the work of men, women do the work of women'. Our culture values highly stratified 'gender' roles. If men are taught that the woman values are weakness, it then furthers that women will be viewed as 'weak' and incompetent of grasping 'masculine' values as we compartmentalize values on the basis of defined 'gender'. We have a patriarchal society, therefore men define what is socially acceptable and what avenues are appropriate for gathering resources financially. Since men do this, the values that men are taught fall directly in line with what is needed to obtain financial resources—a work ideology comprised of a legal-rational system (Weber), autonomy, assertiveness, and competition. Men exclude women from these values and thus the labor market because these values are 'masculine' and that which women cannot not adopt.

The attractiveness of women is defined by Morgan as, "...attractiveness is defined as attractiveness-to-men; women's eroticism is defined as either nonexistent, pathological, or peripheral when it is not directed to phallic goal" (Morgan 2000:151). She proposes that the male-dominated society places itself at the core and that the definition of the periphery can only be found by first understanding the core; essentially, the very definition of every aspect of a woman's life from attractiveness to motherhood is rooted in the functional and working aspects in a male-dominated reality. Women have been taught that their body is a locus of power. They are taught to mold and modify their bodies in order to gain access to prize, position, and power. More importantly, "...affirmation of her beauty brings with it privileged heterosexual affiliation, privileged access to forms of power unavailable to the plain, the ugly, the aged, and the barren" (Morgan 2000:153).

One can argue that women have choice and are autonomous in their right; but I do not agree with this. By getting plastic surgery or other body 'issues', bulimia, anorexia, or any other of the maladies associated with feelings of inadequacy that have come from internalizing unattainable images, the individual consumes the reality that is presented and then constructs their relation to it in their mind. A reality only exists if the reproduction of it and the values assigned to it live in the minds of the collective actors. There has to be agreed upon definitions and concepts amongst the individuals in the masses in order to create a large belief and value system—or framework. If the individual truly did not care about the media images and the patriarchal competition that pits women against each other, then logically there would be none of the problems mentioned above (note that there are numerous counter-culture groups and individuals who do not subscribe to the popular myths knowingly). Morgan sums this up by stating, "…women's public conformity to the norms of beauty often signals a deeper conformity to the norms of compulsive heterosexuality…that what looks like an optimal situation of reflection, deliberation, and self-creating choice often signals conformity at a deeper level" (Morgan 2000:155). I think that people do not believe in the concept of macro-level infusion of cultural control, such as patriarchal oppression and 'beauty', because it is ingrained in us through religious, moral, and social belief that we are unique individuals. I state that cultural controls are so endemic in our reality and daily language that it is difficult for us to separate from them and see the larger forces at work. Part of capitalism marketing rests on the idea that we are special and that we can express ourselves through our consumption choices, but surveys on class show demographics market a specific audience for an economic reason. When I study in the library, I hear different cell phone rings constantly that are songs and jingles from popular media culture; expressing themselves through their individual ring tones only serves to demonstrate that they are cows in the same herd. If you told them this, they would deny it. Their cell phone ring is special and something they chose. Who wants to believe that there exist other forces controlling (maybe influencing is more appropriate) our moves? What could someone do who knew how to harness this knowledge? "Natural destiny is being supplanted by technologically grounded coercion, and the coercion is camouflaged by the language of choice, fulfillment, and liberation" (Morgan 2000:158).

I believe that there is frustration within women because men devalue the values that are assigned to them in our culture. From this frustration comes the awareness and recognition that men have indirectly (and arguably directly) structured society in this way. Thus, men have excluded women from the labor marketplace and have limited their chances for access to financial resources as the 'stigma' of women's values follows the visual master status of being a 'woman'. The alternative, proposed through assimilation processes, is to make the most important day of a woman's life her wedding day and the core of her being the husband and children. This is dichotomous in that there is no balance; the core defines the periphery, and the neglect of 'self' leads to other problems and struggle for a time to feel valued and wanted. Men, on the dichotomous other, center themselves in their universe at work, which is culturally valued in all aspects, and then come home to a family that structures him in the same position.

Of the literature that I have reviewed for this paper on plastic surgery, one theme has become a trend in the qualitative studies—"Women are only doing the best that they can given the limitations that our society has structured for them". If we subscribe to this, then we automatically accept these limitations. We unknowingly buy into the construct that women are objects of adornment and in order to be accepted by 'others', they must alter their bodies to fit the current beauty myth presented and reinforced by the media.

I have never understood what pressure could be so strong that a person would voluntarily alter their body structure to 'fit in' and feel better about themselves. Arguably, plastic surgery combating body image issues is problematic in that the woman who has plastic surgery subscribes to the cultural ideals of beauty, and having this state of mind yields constant dissatisfaction and room for improvement as the same concept fuels capitalism. I ask, "How do women that undergo plastic surgery feel that it will change them both mentally and socially?" As I search for a radical meaning as to why women undergo these surgeries, I believe that there is a biological basis rooted in obtaining resources for social and biological survival.

Gimlin sums up the body in relation to self and presentation best when she states "Because the body is arguably the location from which all social life begins, it is a logical starting point for sociological study. More important, though, the body is a medium of culture" (Gimlin 1995:3). The individual constructs their cultural understanding through the body medium. The individual relates to the culture through the body and the culture relates to the self through the body. We view ourselves (Western culture) as being individuals and being deterministic in our own right and regard. Therefore, the body is an indicator of who the individual is internally and, theoretically, we have free choice as to how we wish to conduct our appearance and ourselves. The gender dichotomy in our culture is expressed through our bodies as well. Traits such as strength and weakness, activity and passivity, and sexuality and neutrality are linked to the physical body. "The very 'nature' of maleness and femaleness is intrinsically embodied" (Gimlin 1995:3).

Appearance is strongly related to personal discipline. We believe that an individual's outward appearance is a reflection of the inner self. We assign value and judge people in regards to their discipline, work ethic, and self-esteem by how they look. If a person is fat we judge them as sloppy and undisciplined. According to Sullivan,

> "He [in regards to Turner 1984] suggests that mass production secularized and transformed the externally imposed moral asceticism of early capitalism into a neo-spartan hedonistic consumerism in which physical appearance is an important cue to internal discipline. Medicine aided this transformation by providing a rational justification for valuing a disciplined, fit body. As a result, the thin, taut, youthful appearance of a fit body became an essential element of the cultural definition of attractiveness" (Sullivan 1993:102).

Who sets the standard in regards to what is considered 'fat' and 'thin'? The definition is strictly cultural and is only in the social context of any given time. The definitions of 'fat' and 'beautiful' have completely changed in the past fifty years; I think that our culture tends to lose sight of that and believes the current cultural mandates on physical appearance to be divine in order. If we did not, then why would people be constantly on 'yo-yo' diets and why is plastic surgery so popular (and rising as an industry annually)? We constantly hear that, in current days, nearly sixty-percent of the population is overweight. If over half of the population in our country is indeed overweight, then we need to recalibrate our working definitions of 'fat' and 'thin'.

In 1954, Miss America was five foot eight inches tall and weighed 132 pounds. Today (2001), she is the same height *but* weighs only 117 pounds. In 1974, the typical fashion model weighed eight percent less than the average woman (according to the Society of the Actuaries). In 1990, the disparity was twenty-three percent. We see that our ideas of 'beauty' in relation to weight, height, and representation in the media have changed significantly over the past fifty years (Gimlin 2001:5). Along with this change is the belief that, "…and women's physical deficiencies (such as unruly hair, cellulite, wrinkled skin, or excess weight) have come increasingly to be viewed as moral weakness. The imperfect body has become a sign of the imperfect character" (Gimlin 2002:5).

I believe the basic ideal of marketing in a capitalistic economy is responsible for influencing women to internalize the body image of the dominant culture which is very selective in the representations that are put forth for consumption. This is analogous to every commodity from stereos to computers; there are *always* 'better' and 'newly improved' products that come out daily. We are told that our owned products are 'outdated' and language is used that implies that they are essentially useless; this is supposed to influence people to purchase or upgrade the new product (that will then be outdated soon). As demonstrated in my previous papers and in the brief example above, the media presents a thinner and more unattainable appearance as time has progressed over the past fifty years, but real American women, according to the Society of the Actuaries, are weighing more. We visually see a graph that is diverging and creating a large gap. Within this gap, all the maladies that are associated with internalization of an unattainable body image reside—bulimia, anorexia nervosa, and low self-esteem. I believe that this internalization influences the desire to change the body in order to fit the images set forth. Gillespie states,

> "But then how do you keep a capitalist consumer culture afloat if people are not kept in a perpetual state of wanting, or feeling insecure? Women—of every ethnic group and color—already programmed to see ourselves as commodities, whose value rises or falls depending on how close or how far we are from some standard of ideal beauty, are the perfect marks" (Gillespie 1993:np).

Plastic surgery has a long history. In 1000 B.C., plastic surgery was reported in India. A person may have their nose cut off for punishment or the husband of an adulterous Hindu wife was reported to have the option of biting off her nose. Procedures that resemble modern day rhinoplasty were developed to restore the noses of the harmed individuals. In the fifteenth century, an Italian physician named Branca performed early rhinoplasty procedures. Techniques for performing plastic surgery have been available for hundreds of years, but the popular use and acceptance has been slow. In 1846, ether and chloroform were discovered. Prior to this, surgeries had to be performed without anesthesia. Patients were at risk of dying from shock and loss of blood; if they did not die on the operating table, infection could soon follow. In 1867, antisepsis was discovered and changed the medical safety of operating room procedures. During this time socially, people generally accepted the idea that the body was the connection between God and human beings. If someone got sick or had an ailment, it was thought to be contributed to immorality. Cosmetic and plastic surgery was thought to disrupt the 'natural order of things' and repair immoral acts that marked the individual. For example, facial surgery was conducted to repair the marks of syphilis, an 'immoral' disease that supposedly came from 'immoral' sexual acts. Medicine became developed as a science in the middle to late 1800's. Surgeons were required to have a university education which separated them from the common practitioner. It was not until the Crimean War did the plastic and reconstructive surgery discipline gain acceptance. Many young men fighting on the front lines were badly injured, burned, and lost appendages. Plastic surgeons brought their work to the front lines of the war and made great strides for the profession. Socially, the surgeons were viewed as people helping the young, brave men who were fighting the war (Davis 1995:14-17).

"Cosmetic surgery stands, for many theorists and social critics, as the ultimate symbol of invasion of the human body for the sake of physical beauty. It has epitomized for many—including myself—the astounding lengths to which contemporary women will go in order to obtain bodies that meet the current ideals of attractiveness" (Gimlin 1995: 78). Cosmetic surgery is the fastest growing specialty in medicine. "Unlike other surgical procedures, the risks are not weighed against the potential for improved physical function or reduced deviant appearance due to congenital malformation, trauma or previous surgical mutilation such as mastectomy. Instead, the risks of cosmetic surgery are weighed solely against the value of a more attractive appearance" (Sullivan 1993:98). Medicine has a social mandate to improve the health and physical well being of the general population. It is contradictory for the medical community to perform cosmetic procedures at the risk of physical health as any number of problems could arise from the surgery. Sullivan suggests that medicalization can occur whenever physicians can serve the interests of their patients and serve their own political and economic interests.

Women undergo cosmetic surgery for a variety of reasons. On a macro level, I argue that it is because a body image has been internalized in such a way that the individual believes that they will be denied access to resources, such as position and prestige, if they do not modify their physical being to meet the prescribed standard. Morgan gives three reasons of her own (micro level):

1. "Electing to undergo the surgery necessary to create youth and beauty artificially not only appears to but often actually does give a woman a sense of identity that, to some extent, she has chosen herself.

2. It offers her the potential to raise her status both socially and economically by increasing her opportunities for heterosexual affiliation (especially with white men).

3. By committing herself to the pursuit of beauty, a woman integrates her life with a consistent set of values and choices that bring her widespread approval and a resulting sense of increased self-esteem" (Morgan 2000:153).

The number of cosmetic medical procedures reported by board-certified plastic surgeons increased sixty-three percent between 1981 and 1988. Liposuction was introduced in the United States in 1982 and became the most frequent procedure by 1988. New techniques and procedures for breast implants, forehead lifts, injections of fat and use of Retin-A to gradually peel superficial wrinkled skin emerged in the 1980's as well. The frequencies of procedures is much higher than the numbers reported by the board-certified surgeons because members of two other American Board of Medical Services—dermatology and ophthalmology—routinely do cosmetic procedures in their areas of expertise (Sullivan 1993).

Gender and class both play an important part in legitimizing a medical approach to aesthetic surgery. Surgeons and patients see cosmetic surgery as 'normal' for women. It is 'natural' for them to be concerned with their appearance (Dull and West 1991). In 1993, eighty-four percent of cosmetic surgeries were performed on women (Sullivan 1993:99). In 1987, women in the United States had 94,000 breast implant surgeries, 85,000 eyelid surgeries, 82,000 nose jobs, 73,230 liposuctions, and 67,000 face lifts (Gimlin 1995:79). As of 1995, three hundred million dollars are spent every year on cosmetic surgery and the amount is increasing annually by ten percent (Gimlin 2000:78). In 2001, 13 million Americans spent a total of 7 billion dollars on cosmetic surgery, both surgical and non-surgical (www.plasticsurgery.org). A random sample of 560 cosmetic surgery patients conducted by the American Society of Plastic and Reconstructive Surgeons in 1989 revealed that most that undergo procedures are from the middle and upper classes. Over four-fifths have some college education and fifty-eight percent had some sort of graduate education. Of note, two-fifths of full facelift patients are under fifty as are half or more of those having eyelifts, forehead lifts, and chemical peels (Sullivan 1993). The average age of a woman getting breast implants is thirty-six years and has two children (Nader 1997:716). As the research demonstrates, the individual undergoing plastic surgery is (in demographic) disproportionately a woman in the middle to upper class within a certain age range.

"That we are surrounded by homogenizing and normalizing images—images whose content is far from arbitrary, but instead suffused with the dominance of gendered, racial, class, and other cultural iconography—seems so obvious as to be almost embarrassing to be arguing here" (Bordo 1990:657). In Western society, we have an entrenched belief stating that the individual is responsible for 'making it happen'. 'It' can be anything from education to a 'perfect' body. We hold the individual responsible for his/her actions *and* for his/her failures. Our culture values a thin figure, so any deviation is considered a 'failure' physically which means a failure personally. Bordo discusses many examples of advertisements that place this responsibility on the individual. Many of them depict thin, muscular men and 'beautiful' women enjoying a particular product with the ad slogan endowing the reader with the empowerment to consciously 'choose' this body—"All the right equipment (with a muscular woman and depicted and phrases describing her muscular success)" for a gym advertisement and "If you could choose your own body, which would you choose?" showing women working out in a gym while drinking Evian water. The advertisements disproportionately featured white people as the models for the product. The ad that featured a black woman was that for contact lenses. The slogan for this product is, "Eyes as brown as violets?" The advertisement has a dark-skinned woman with violets in her hair as the ad center focus is on her eyes. The function of the product is to lighten the color of brown eyes, alluding to achieving a blue color ultimately. The television commercial stated, "DuraSoft colored contact lenses: Get brown eyes a second look". A trend we see is the representation of 'beauty' being aligned with white, middle to upper class values of thinness reflecting inner character and individual determinism (Bordo 1990:654-59). This also happens to be the long blond haired, blue-eyed 'beauty' such as Christie Brinkley of the 1980's or Jennifer McCarthy of the 1990's. Bordo then discusses a *Donahue* show where advertisements and products that are aimed at ethnic people in order to 'normalize' them to the prevailing cultural idea of beauty (these products would be the mentioned contact lenses and curling irons used to straighten hair). "The question posed by Donahue: Is this ad racist? Donahue clearly thought there was a controversy to be stirred up here, for he stocked his audience full of women of color and white women to discuss the implications of the ad. But Donahue, apparently, was living in a different decade than most of his audience, who found nothing 'wrong' with the ad, and everything 'wrong' with any inclinations to 'make it a political question'" (Bordo 1990:657-58).

"Most noticeably, the ethnic composition of consumers has changed so that in recent years there are more racial and ethnic minorities. In 1994, 14% of cosmetic surgery patients were Latinos, African Americans, and Asian Americans [according to the American Society of Plastic and Reconstructive Surgeries]" (Kaw 1993) [brackets added]. Women are the majority consumers of cosmetic surgery across all racial and ethnic groups. Kaw states that Asian women are motivated by the same reasons as white women to undergo surgery—which is the desire to look their best—but furthers that white women do not opt for surgeries that are markers of racial identity as Asian women do. This means that the most popular procedures for white women are liposuction, breast augmentation, and wrinkle removal procedures whereas for Asian women they are "double eyelid" surgery and surgical scalping of the nose tip. "Double eyelid" surgery is a procedure where folds of skin are excised from the upper eyelids to create a crease above each eye that makes the eye appear wider. The surgical scalping of the nose is to give a more "chiseled" appearance and usually this is achieved by implanting silicone or cartilage in the bridge of the nose and then sculpting it and, for appearance purposes, "…'westernizing' of their own eyes and the creation of higher noses in hopes of better job and marital prospects" (Morgan 2000:155). Kaw furthers that Asian women in her study underwent these procedures because they had internalized a body image produced by the dominant culture's racial ideology. Once internalized, they begin to dislike their biological racial characteristics and thus wish to change the parts of their bodies that are the clearest indicators of their race (Kaw 1993). It is not only Asian women whose choose procedures that are to modify racially identified features. Morgan states that black women buy toxic bleaching agents in hopes to attain lighter skin. "What is being created in all of these instances is not simply beautiful bodies and faces but white, Western, Anglo-Saxon bodies in a racist, anti-Semitic context" (Morgan 2000:155).

One of the main criticisms of plastic surgery is the dangers involved in many of the procedures. It is painful and risky; each operation possesses its own set of risks. Pain, numbness, and discoloration can follow liposuction; this can linger for up to six months following the surgery. The most serious disabilities include blood clots, liquid depletion, and even death. Women who undergo breast augmentation have a thirty to fifty percent chance of suffering from some side effects that include painful swelling of the breasts, loss of feeling in the nipple, and hardening of the breasts (Gimlin 1995:79).

Another criticism of cosmetic surgery is the focus on the implications of such procedures for "contemporary conceptualizations of the body and identity." In modern times with modern procedures and technology, the body is seen as having limitless change. The body, instead of a dysfunctional object requiring medical intervention, becomes a commodity like a car or a house; it is something to be bought and sold which defines the inner character of the possessor. "The body is a symbol of selfhood, but its relation to its inhabitant is shaped primarily by the individual's capacity for material consumption" (Gimlin 1995:80).

Gimlin would fully disagree with the idea that I propose in this paper that, ultimately, women are not sovereign decision-makers in subscription to the beauty myth as they undergo plastic surgery. She takes the approach and agrees with the individual choice of women while they know the risks and cultural pressures involved. She conducted interviews with twenty women who were in the process of undergoing plastic surgery procedures at a clinic in Long Island. The women were having different types of cosmetic surgery and represented many different races and ethnicities. Many argue that it is the mindset of continually finding fault with one's personal appearance that will lead to multiple cosmetic surgeries as one flaw is found after one is corrected. Gimlin states that this is a misconception and that in her research she found that plastic surgery often achieves the goals intended by the client (Gimlin 2000).

Gimlin does agree with the division of race, class, and ethnicity in regards to the procedure chosen. Asian women have their eyes reshaped, Jewish and Italian women have rhinoplasty in order to 'correct' ethnically identifiable features. Gimlin further states that critics of plastic surgery fail to explore the complicated process that women undergo to integrate the procedure into their identity. She states

> "If not in feminist theory, then in popular culture, there lies an implicit notion that the benefits of plastic surgery are somehow inauthentic and, therefore, undeserved. Although the critics of plastic surgery are insistent that appearance should not be the measure of a woman's worth, the women who have plastic surgery are nonetheless participants in a culture in which appearance is often taken as an expression of inner state" (Gimlin 2000:81).

When Gimlin studied women in aerobics classes, she concluded that they were working to *detach* their identities from their bodies whereas with plastic surgery women are trying to *reattach* their bodies to their identities. They are using the procedure to tell a story about their bodies, yet must also find a way to demonstrate that the new look is deserved in order to mitigate the criticisms of it being inauthentic. "She is unhappy with her appearance. But she must also defend herself for the very efforts she makes to alter that appearance" (Gimlin 2000:81).

Gimlin mediates between the sovereignty of women to choose their appearance and the cultural representations that give us a reality on which to set a standard to. She argues that plastic surgery does work for the women who choose to undergo it, but only in the context of the culture of appearance "…that is highly restrictive and which is less a culture of beauty than it is a system of control based on the physical representations of gender, age, and ethnicity" (Gimlin 2000:89).

I disagree with what Gimlin concludes in regards to personal choice versus the hypodermic model. She states

> "To be sure, the women's decisions to undergo surgery were shaped by broader cultural considerations—by notions of what constitutes beauty, by

distinctively ethnic notions of beauty…by the assumption that a woman's worth is measured by her appearance. Yet to portray women I talked to as some sort of 'cultural dopes', tossed and battered by cultural forces beyond their understanding, as passively submitting to the demands of beauty, is to badly misrepresent them" (Gimlin 2000:96).

I think that Gimlin is missing the root of her own argument here and contradicts herself. She recognizes that the women that underwent surgery were influenced by 'broader cultural considerations'. This *does* make them 'cultural dopes' and the women choosing to undergo cosmetic surgery *does* make them 'tossed and battered by cultural forces beyond their understanding'. I do not differentiate between levels of consciousness of an individual when the subscription to particular aspects of popular culture has been made. This instance is a perfect example and the logic is very simple: Women who are choosing to undergo plastic surgery are doing so because they feel inadequate or 'flawed' in some aesthetic capacity (entirely born out of culture), which means that the woman is basing her physical value in the definitions given by popular culture. This definition is defined primarily by the media, consumed by individuals, and then fed back to others. It is a vicious cycle, a tornado-like whirlwind. The agenda of the media is to make money and sell products to consumers, so the beauty images presented are the ones that are consumed by the masses in large numbers (as consumer dollars directs the agenda) and become the standard for the masses to unknowingly subscribe to. When I state that consumer dollars drive the agenda, then it is premised on the belief that consumers 'vote' for the images in the media and the images must be what the consumer wants as majority rule. I am not refuting this argument. I am attempting to explain a macro-level agenda that the masses are not aware of or of their constant participation in it. Our 'menu' has centered on a particular beauty type for nearly two generations now, and it would take massive social and media change to undo the prevailing beauty myth. It is possible, but it would take an upheaval of the entire industry.

It does not matter if the woman is aware of what cultural forces are pressuring her to conform; the bottom line is that she *does* conform by undergoing the surgery. It is inconsequential to say that the woman is 'doing the best she can given the restrictions'; I believe this is an excuse to passively participate and perpetuate the unknown degradation. I understand that we all have to socially survive given the parameters of our culture, but trying to speak of rational choice and sovereignty in a situation that is based in the unconscious subscription to cultural forces *is nothing more* than another way to give permission for the individual to be fooled about both their own importance in the masses and the manipulation they are succumbing to. This is marketing in capitalism—let the consumer believe that their consumption choices are unique in how they define themselves; that makes it easier to herd them to slaughterhouse cathedral of our modern quasi-religion called materialism.

In conclusion, I have addressed many different arguments that all come together under the umbrella of 'resources'. We are biologically disposed to have sexual drives. I argue that we are biologically disposed to mate. We want to ensure the safety and future for our offspring; whether we choose a mate that has rocks tall enough so that the ground will not freeze the clutch or the mate that has financial resources to guarantee life without hardship, the choices are made through a system of cognitive evaluations that achieves the goal *given the options for survival.* Just as penguins and squirrels have found ways to adapt in order to ensure that this goal is achieved, we find avenues that allow us to given the social structure of our culture that is primarily based on a system of rewards and punishments. In current times, cosmetic surgery is a 'leveler' and allows women to compete for title of 'alpha female', just as Livia and Effie did. Watching 'Joe Millionaire' last night demonstrates my point precisely—there are currently only three women left vying for his acceptance, and they are each planting unkind words and rumors about each other to 'Joe'. Two of the three had breast enlargements prior to coming on the show (not specifically to go on the show). Also, the monogamous dates they are taking turns going on with 'Joe' have turned sexual, with the female always instigating the first advance. Are these actions competition for the resources of a millionaire? Maybe I am wrong—they could sincerely love him…

Women undergoing cosmetic surgery are trying to adapt to a 'beauty myth' and thus compete for the limited resource of the most socially adapted men. The penguin with the tallest rock stack can choose which female he wants to mate with—he has options. Women that come closer to achieving the 'unattainable body' have more options as well. These women can then select a mate based on the criteria that they choose, which for most that undergo cosmetic surgery (life based on superficiality) will be money, power, and prestige.

What is the 'Perfect' Female Physique and Who is Defining It?

"Drunks, gluttons, smokers, and sedentaries (now derisively called 'couch potatoes' in the new perjorative of healthism) are viewed as an inferior class of people, certainly unfit, undependable, inefficient and probably unclean in mind and spirit as well as body" (Edgely and Brissett 1990:263).

I argue that the 'beauty image' of women that is presented by our media is a social problem. Best gives a workable definition of a social problem by quoting Farely who states, "A social problem, then, can be defined as a condition that: (1) is widely regarded as undesirable or as a source of difficulties; (2) is caused by the actions or inactions of people or of a society; [and] (3) affects or is thought to affect a large number of people" (Best 1995:3). I use the Health Nazi article by Edgley and Brissett (1990) as a frame of structure. Many of the theories and ideas that they propose are very similar to the 'beauty image' because they primarily hold the individual responsible for their achievements and failures as well as use this as a means to divert attention from the social pressures or 'matrix' that is truly responsible. The article traces the social framework that gives legitimation to the health industry and I compare this to how the media constructs the 'beauty myth' and gives legitimization to it in the same manner. Finally, I will use research data to provide an answer to the question, "What is the perfect body for women, according to the media?"

In a 1986 Gallup Poll, ninety-three percent of Americans agreed with the following statement: "If I take the right actions, I can stay healthy". In recent times, there has been a cultural explosion of health programs marketed in our country. Among many examples, health food stores, spas, personal trainers, television channels, scientific research, department stores, and dieting programs have emerged as a response to the 'health craze'. They are marketing health through individual achievement; this is important because the health industry has placed the ultimate responsibility of health on the individual, thus negating the numerous factors that influence health such as genetics and socioeconomic status (Edgley and Brissett 1990).

Edgley and Brissett quote Stein by stating, "…[Stein] notes that the promotion of a 'wellness' ideology not only treats complex human problems simplistically (e.g. running as a cure for depression; exercise for smoking cessation), but diverts attention from pressing social issues by pre-occupying each person with his own individual well-being" (Edgley and Brissett 1990:258). When we have constructed the ideal 'beauty type' through various avenues of the media, we have a standard to judge ourselves by and a place for us to start evaluation. The problem is that this ideal is unattainable. The images are consumed and then believed to be the standard. I do not believe that the majority of women understand that these images change as the social tides do, and that the internalization of them is key in selling products to the consumers of these images. McKinely and Hyde believe that women "internalize cultural body standards so that the standards appear to originate from the self and believe that achieving these standards is possible even in the face of considerable evidence to the contrary" (McKinley and Hyde 1996:183). Just as we place the responsibility of a 'good' and 'physically fit' body on the individual's achievement and efforts, our culture places the responsibility of adhering to the 'beauty' myth' on women in the same fashion. By doing this, there exist women who subscribe to this belief that berate themselves for not looking a 'certain' way; hence the proliferation of plastic and cosmetic surgery from the mid 1980's until recent times (as well as the health 'craze'). In 2001, 13 million Americans spent a total of 7 billion dollars on cosmetic surgery, both surgical and non-surgical (www.plasticsurgery.org). We also see the health industry exploding around us in industry growth, and all of these programs also ultimately place the responsibility on the individual. In accordance with what Stein states, I must agree that this is only a diversion from the social pressures that are truly influencing us to conform to the ideal. If an individual is preoccupied with their personal appearance and performance, what would be gained by questioning and thus destabilizing the base of the social pressures at work? When individuals are ignorant to the social pressures, Russell Jacoby calls this "'the permanent emergency of the individual,' and its consequent ignorance of the social matrix in which all such movements are imbedded" (Edgley and Brissett 1990:259). The 'emergency' is the constant and instant need to fix what is 'wrong', which is truly only defined by the social matrix in which these messages are embedded.

Self-righteous intolerance is the base of the health and 'beauty image' movements. Our culture sends messages that anyone, with proper exercise, diet, and attitude can be healthy and have a good physical look. If people do not do this, they are seen as deviant. It is difficult for subscribers to the health movement to fathom why someone would choose not to take part, when they, in fact, *should*. Once again, we see the repetition of choice in regards to these two movements. We attach this 'deviance' to an imperfect character as our culture attaches outward body appearance to inner traits and disposition (Edgely and Brissett 1990). Appearance is strongly related to personal discipline in our culture. We believe that a person's physical appearance is a reflection of the inner self. We assign value and judge someone as sloppy and undisciplined if they are 'fat'. Our culture changes 'beauty images' as the times change. For example, in 1954 Miss America was five foot eight inches tall and weighed 132 pounds. Today (2001), she is the same height but weighs only 117 pounds. In 1974, the typical fashion model weighed eight percent less than the average woman (according to the Society of the Actuaries). In 1990, the disparity was twenty-three percent. We see that our ideas of 'beauty' in relation to weight, height, and representation in the media have changed significantly over the past fifty years (Gimlin 2001:5). Along with this change is the belief that, "…and women's physical deficiencies (such as unruly hair, cellulite, wrinkled skin, or excess weight) have come increasingly to be viewed as moral weakness. The imperfect body has become a sign of the imperfect character" (Gimlin 2002:5).

Edgley and Brisset use the term 'Health Nazi' as a way to describe the condition of self-righteousness driving the health-crazed individuals. They use this term because, "…Nazism showed how the restoration and repair of the social body and that of the physical body were indistinguishable. The elimination of evil within—often in the metaphor of cancer—was a precondition to the attainment of inner unity, harmony, integrity, health, and will. Health could only be restored by eradicating the disease—those people whose very existence symbolized decadence and death" (Edgley and Brissett 1990:260). Our culture believes and perpetuates this same idea, therefore I will now use the term 'Body Nazi'. The 'disease' is the fat that plagues the bodies of women and, according to the mandate given by the Body Nazis, *should* be eliminated (since all *can* with proper measures taken). Once all of the fat is lost, the woman must have a large bust and narrow hips. Genetics can be fixed by plastic and cosmetic surgery, so once again all women *can*.

According to Edgley and Brissett, the 'perfect' body is

> "It is slender, fit, and glowing. It does not smoke. If it drinks, it does so in moderation. It carefully regulates its diet in terms of calories, carbohydrates,

fats, salts, and sugar. It exercises regularly and intensely. It showers (not bathes) frequently. It engages only in safe sex. It sleeps regular hours. It has the correct amount of body fat (women 20%; men 15%). It has flexibility…it has proper muscle strength…it has appropriate aerobic capacity…in short, the perfect body is one that is biochemically, physiologically, and autonomically sound" (Edgley and Brissett 1990:262).

The perfect body for a woman (according to those making claims in the media) in regards to physical shape, is "the perfect ten", that is a ten-inch differentiation between breast, waist, and hip measurements. In current times, the ideal is 36-24-36, 5'4 in height, and 115 pounds.

There are social and personal rewards that allegedly come from having a healthy body both internally and outwardly. Better relationships both in work and personal life will ensue, more energy, more work achievement, and inclusion into the 'elite' as a Body Nazi are all rewards. In advertising throughout the mid to late 1900's, women that fit the 'beauty image' of the given time where shown to be financially successful (Marchand 1985). We rarely see 'obese' women or those that are 'out of control' of their bodies in advertisements depicting successful women. "Furthermore, for North American women, higher social class is strongly related to thinness and dieting" (Garner et. al. 1980:483). To attain this unattainable ideal, people are driven to moderation and control over all things that have been deemed unhealthy (Edgely and Brissett 1990).

The rewards of attaining the 'perfect body' are more than simply physical and personal. Our culture has spun the meaning into a spiritual entity. I would argue that the health craze has become somewhat of a quasi-religion in our country. The cathedrals are health clubs, religious texts are health products utilized to perfect the body, and the holy figureheads (preachers, priests) are the infomercial 'experts' promising spiritual salvation through use of the new product that will ensure the weight loss and ideal shaping of the consumer. "The body is conceived of as a temple of God, secularly translated as 'health', and through a multitude of self-denials and resistances to temptation, both the body and the spirit are strengthened" (Edgely and Brissett 1990:267).

Garner et. al. (1980) conducted a study comparing the height, weight, bust, and hips of *Playboy* centerfolds. They did the same with contestants of the Miss America pageant. *Playboy* magazine allowed the research team to recover the height, weight, and body measurements of all 240 monthly playmates which appeared from 1959-1978. The average age, height, weight, bust, waist, and hip measurements from 1959-1978 are presented in the writing. The averages, in total, are five feet, five inches in height, 116 pounds, thirty-six inch bust, twenty-three inch waist, and thirty-five inch hips. "In addition, the average weight of the playmates was compared to population means reported by the 1959-1978 Society of Actuaries" (Garner et. al. 1980:484). With each respective year, the average measurements of that year in *Playboy* were compared against the Society of the Actuaries measurements. The yearly mean weight for the centerfolds was significantly less than the corresponding population mean. The changes within the playmates over the twenty-year time period is most important: "While absolute weight did not decline because heights were increasing, a regression analysis showed that the percent of average weight for age and height decreased significantly over the 20 yr [sic]. These absolute declines in measurements occurred in women who were increasing in height" (Garner et. al 1980:485). In 1968, the playmates had the weight lowest in regards to the population mean. We see, through this study, that the height of the playmate increased while her weight decreased along with the playmate weight being significantly lower than the women's mean population weight.

Height, weight, and age data were derived for both the winners and the contestants of the Miss America Pageant from 1959 through 1978. The means were calculated and, once again, compared to the means reported by the 1959 Society of Actuaries. The averages, from 1959 to 1978, are five foot, four and one-half inches, thirty-six inch bust, a twenty-three inch waist, and thirty-six inch hips. Garner et. al. (1980) found that contestants declined yearly in weight by .28 pounds and the winners declined yearly in weight by .37 pounds. Average height in both winners and contestants drastically jumped (two inches) from 1968 to 1970, along with average waist size increasing two inches from 1960 to 1978.

From the above data, we can average the averages of the two studies. The average studied woman is five foot, four and three quarters of an inch tall, 116 pounds (*Playboy* data being used), thirty-six inch bust, twenty-three inch waist, and thirty-five and a half inch hips. In comparing the two studies, there is very little difference between the two averages; in fact, they are exactly correlated within less than one-half an inch. The 'ideal beauty' should have a ratio of 1.3 between her bust and waist. The average waist is twenty-three inches. That would make the 'ideal' bust right at thirty inches. Given the studies of the *Playboy* centerfolds and the Miss America Pageant winners, the ratio would be close to 1.5. This is comparable to the 'curvaceous' look of 1917 and then the 1940's when looking at the graph of bust-to-waist ratios in their content analysis study (Garner et. al. 1980).

We see, through research data collected, that the 'beauty image' gaining reward in the media is unattainable as it is compared to the data from the Society of Actuaries. I believe that this image is consumed by women. After consumed, this imaged can influence eating disorders, the health 'craze', and cosmetic/plastic surgery as the quest for the unattainable body begins. We see that the health 'craze' ideology has been consumed by participants and then reified through many claims, such as attaching inner character to outer appearance and passing value-laden judgments against those that choose to not participate.

What Institutions Have Emerged to Combat the Obesity Plague and Provide Products for Aesthetic Enhancement?

"It's true that obesity contributes to diabetes, heart disease, arthritis and some types of cancer" (Hellmich 2002:1D).

"…'claims express demand in a moral universe…just as there are vocabularies of motives, so there may be a wide choice of values that may be used to articulate a claim" (Spencer quoting Spector and Kistuse 1977:93)

The above quote was written by Nancy Hellmich, a columnist for the 'Life' section of the popular newspaper *USA TODAY*. She is a claims-maker. *USA TODAY* is a nation-wide newspaper that millions rely on daily to receive the news. When writers such as Nancy Hellmich make claims like the above quote, people believe them and they become a reality. Why would we doubt her facts or validity? She works for *USA TODAY*. This blind belief in perceived authority pervades our culture and gives rise to claims-making institutions. These same institutions create and perpetuate the social problem of obesity as they both attempt to inform and remedy it. I am going to be using media sources as my examples in this paper. The mass media is the manner in which most citizens are informed. Using media examples to demonstrate how obesity has been constructed as a problem—along with the institutions that have emerged to 'fix' it—is the only way to effectively categorize and analyze the situation.

Obesity is seen as an individual choice. In the previous chapters, I discussed how our culture has made inner character and outward appearance inseparable. Social pressures and individual genetics are not taken into account; claims-makers give blanket statements that are applicable to all. The most notable is the manner in which the problem of obesity has been constructed by our culture and the social institutions that have risen to 'combat' the problem. I use the term 'combat' because many claims-makers commonly use this metaphor. According to Spencer, Best states that claimants are aware that declaring 'war' on a social problem "appropriates the image of an enemy that is evil (Best 1999, pp. 145-147) and menacing (Gorelick 1989, p. 429) as well as an image of 'us' against 'it' (or perhaps 'them')" (Spencer 2000:32-33). Numerous 'experts' have emerged after having conducted studies that link obesity to various health ailments, primary heart disease and type two diabetes. For example, "The North American Association for Study of Obesity (NAASO) is a leading scientific society dedicated to the study of obesity. NAASO is committed to encouraging research on the causes, treatment, and prevention of obesity, and to keeping the scientific community and public informed of new advances in the field" (www.naaso.org). "The American Obesity Association is a non-profit advocacy organization founded in 1995 whose fundamental mission is to have obesity regarded as a disease of epidemic proportions. AOA is composed of lay persons, professional providers and industry supporters (www.obesity.org). As obesity is demonized and categorized further as a social problem, we have seen a whole industry spawn that has taken on a life of its own. In this chapter, I am going to identify and discuss some of the claims-makers that are giving legitimization to the obesity problem. I am also going to talk about social institutions that have evolved as a manner of dealing with this social problem. Finally, I am going to discuss companies that have emerged that neither deal with obesity nor health, but rather provide physically-altering products meant to morph particular body parts into 'desirable' by popular culture.

The National Institute of Health estimates that 39.8 million adults, representing 22.3% of the nation's population over age 20, are obese. The NIH defines obesity as having a body mass index [BMI] (a ratio of weight to height) of 30 or more. Morbid obesity is defined as having a BMI of 40 or more. The Department of Health and Human Services estimates that obesity results in approximately 300,000 deaths each year; only smoking causes more preventable deaths annually in the United States. The Surgeon General estimates that the public health costs attributable to being overweight and obesity now come to about 117 billion a year, whereas smoking is 140 billion (Parloff 2002:53). Obesity plays a role in other chronic health conditions. Watson Wyatt Worldwide estimates, for example, that of the $2.4 billion spent annually on medical costs for type 2 diabetes, 61% is attributable to obesity. Nearly 25% of the $57 million spent annually on osteoarthritis and 17% of the $1.6 billion spent annually on hypertension are attributable to obesity. Obesity has reached epidemic proportions, according to the U.S. Centers for Disease Control. The CDC found that, from 1991 to 2000, the number of obese Americans rose 61%. In fact, rates of obesity (being 30 pounds or more over ideal body weight) increased from 12 percent in 1991 to nearly 18 percent in 1998. Just as alarming, the number of Americans with diabetes rose 49% during the same time period, according to the CDC. We are now in the midst of fighting a 'Fat Plague' (Financial News 2001; Hanlon 2003; Hellmich 2002; Roberts 2002; University Wire 2001).

Obesity is not seen as a disease by the medical community. Therefore, prescription diet pills are not covered by health providers. The nation's leading obesity organizations are pushing to change that. They state obesity is a disease that needs medical intervention and should be covered by insurance, HMOs, and Medicare and Medicaid. They argue that more people would seek help if it were covered, and they say that even modest weight loss of as little as 5% produces health benefits such as lowering blood pressure and blood sugar as well as improving cholesterol levels. And they argue that those changes may save health care costs in the long run. Others argue that treating obesity would cost too much and would substantially raise health care premiums for companies and individuals. They argue that even if people lost weight, there is no guarantee they would keep it off (Hellmich 2002; University Wire 2001).

Obesity is not only seen as a personal problem, but also viewed as a financial burden for employers. In light of the research and findings being produced concerning obesity, many national companies have instituted health and exercise plans for their employees. Union Pacific Railroad devoted 2 million dollars last year [2001] to 'health'. They have gone as far as to allow their staff physician, Dennis Richling, the authority to give 150 obese employees the diet drug Meridia. They claim that the steps they have taken are saving them 50 million dollars a year in medical costs (Parloff 2002). They are not alone. General Motors and Coors Brewing Company have similar plans aimed at reducing employee weight in hopes to curve health care costs that result from such a chosen lifestyle (Hellmich 2002).

Fortune magazine printed an article titled, "Is Fat the Next Tobacco?" This article compares lawsuits that have recently been brought against fast-food companies to those won against the tobacco industry. The argument against tobacco is that smoking is addictive and from that addiction, over a series of years, come smoking-related illnesses. Tobacco companies were proven to know that their products were addictive and that they caused health problems. The argument against food companies is that the rates of overweight and obese among small children have doubled since 1980. Rates among adolescents have tripled. Lawyers claim that food companies know that their products are unhealthy and are aggressively marketing children/adolescents. In 1999, physicians began reporting an alarming rise in children of obesity-linked type 2 diabetes. Once a young person develops this disease, they will never get rid of it. Smoking addiction is irreversible (Parloff 2002).

Basically, all of the above mentioned examples are claims-makers stating a social problem that now exists. The problem is embedded in the matrix of our media; it exists all around us with consensus from one source to the next that *something must be done about it*. After the problem has been identified, solutions are proposed. What institutions have emerged to 'deal' with the obesity and weight problem that our country is facing?

The diet industry is a multibillion dollar enterprise in our country, making about 30 billion dollars in 1990 (Epstein and Thompson 194:10). The biggest names in the diet industry are Jenny Craig (born in 1983), Weight Watchers (born in 1963), and Nutri/System. Since 1963, more than 25 million people have joined Weight Watchers (Torrens 1998:31). Diet centers primarily use anecdotal advertising. The success stories are heightened (yet always with a disclaimer at the bottom of the ad stating 'results not typical'), therefore the failure rates are masked. This gives the individual hope. "The average weight loss client is a female, between 35 and 50, competent at a chosen profession whether inside the home or outside, with self-esteem closely tied to numbers on the scale" (Epstein and Thompson 1994:61). Losing twenty pounds at Nutri/System can cost more than 1,000 dollars (Epstein and Thompson 1994:21).

In researching and comparing/contrasting institutions that have emerged to help people fight obesity with a product, I noticed similarities. Unless otherwise noted, all of the websites showcased white women that appear to be in the middle class [this research was conducted in 2003]. They fit the 'soccer mom' profile (being 30ish with 'other burdening responsibilities'). Jenny Craig had two minorities, and Metabolife had one man. All the websites offered success stories, weight loss suggestions, and eating tips.

Jenny Craig promotes 'healthy' living through their diet plans. The goals of their program are 1.) A healthy approach with food 2.) An active lifestyle and 3.) A balanced approach to living. The program goals are ultimately aimed toward "…helps clients learn how to eat the foods they want, increase their energy level through simple activity, and build more balance into their lives for optimal weight loss and well-being" (http://www.jennycraig.com/programs/faq-pi.asp). The company states that they aim at teaching individuals how to maintain weight loss once the program is complete. This can be done by continuing to pay for the services and speaking weekly to a 'trained' counselor. They offer food, that the consumer must purchase separately in addition to the plan, that "…by following the Jenny Craig Menus, you'll be practicing habits like portion control that are essential for healthy weight loss and successful weight management" (http://www.jennycraig.com/programs/faq-pi.asp). From the goals to pitch to purchase their specific food line, the base premise is that the individual is responsible for their actions and Jenny Craig can help you lasso the out-of-control behavior, called over-eating, that the individual needs help with.

Weight Watchers (www.weightwatchers.com) appears to have a somewhat similar philosophy as Jenny Craig, but a different way to sell their product. Their philosophy is the same in goals and weight loss maintenance, but differs in that they take a 'scientific' approach to weight loss. Weight Watchers aims to teach people how to eat normal foods, but under a calculated/managed program. The system rests on points. Points are calculated via a calculator that can be accessed by paying members. Food items, as well as information from nutrition labels, are used in the calculation. Recipes are available for free online, and members get counseling groups to attend weekly. There are comprehensive guides on how to handle food and not break 'points' in every eating situation, from upcoming holidays to eating out. The website pictures white, middle to upper class women (same as Jenny Craig). I saw a few men in the pictures while navigating, but they were in the foreground as accessories to the women. The philosophy also includes men in the wordage, which was uncommon in my research.

Not only are diet programs popular, but so are the diet pills. These pills are meant to suppress the appetite. Ideally, if a person is not hungry then they will not eat. One of the most popular is Dexatrim—"natural weight loss for a healthy lifestyle" (www.dexatrim.com). Dexatrim offers very brief suggestions for meals and exercise. When I first opened the website, a 'diet tip of the month' was the first item that I noticed. It stated that "Any serving of food bigger than your fist or a bar of soap is too big!" The website states that the product is a balance between vitamins and weight loss/fat burning minerals. Overall, the website was not that informative or comprehensive.

Metabolife took our country by storm in 2000. The product is now the fastest selling weight management product in our country (www.metabolife.com). The producers claim that "…used by millions of Americans to fight another battle, those excessive pounds of fat brought on by overeating and lack of exercise.* By raising a user's metabolism, this herbal formula not only causes a more energetic feeling, but reduces the appetite and helps the body more rapidly burn the calories that it does take in.*" (http://www.metabolife.com/about/history.htm) [note that the asterisks indicate that the statements have not been approved by the Food and Drug Administration]. The product is hugely successful because it contains Ephedra, a herb traditionally used in China for asthma relief and athletic enhancement. It has also been linked to cause seizures, heart attacks, and strokes. Ephedra is used in most dietary supplements, but Metabolife was using an amount above the FDA's recommendations. That is why the FDA did not approve the product originally, and why lawsuits plagued the company through last year [2002]. Metabolife International lost a 4.1 million dollar lawsuit in 2002, and has since received negative press. They were ordered to pay this amount to four people who claimed that they suffered strokes from the diet product. Now, there is an 'Ephedra Scare' in the health industry that has led competing brands to market Ephedra-free products, such as Dexatrim (Marsa 2002, Redfearn 2003, Roan 2002).

Pills are not only seen as the magic beans that melt away the fat, but also are constructed as an alternative to cosmetic surgery. Along with the construction of 'fat' as a social problem, an industry of aesthetic value has emerged. We know that plastic surgery has grown to be a billion dollar business since the 1980's. The second most popular cosmetic surgery is breast enhancement. What is someone supposed to do that is unhappy with their breast appearance, yet refuses (or does not have the money) to undergo cosmetic surgery? Since the late 1980's, numerous 'breast enhancing' pills and creams have come to the market as viable solutions. The most popular, Bloussant, claims "The all-natural breast enhancement, gradually augment the size and shape of your breasts using a formula that promotes a healthy transformation. "With Bloussant breast enhancement, adding inches to your bust is now a less expensive alternative to costly surgery" (www.wellquestintl.com). Naturally, testimonials are given. Many breast-enhancing creams are available as well. There are literally hundreds of competing companies, such as Natural Firm (www.naturalfirm.com), Natural Breast (www.naturalbreast.com), and Small Breast Solutions (www. smallbreastsolutions.com). The difference between the pills and the cream (as claimed by the companies) is that the pills 'target' the fatty tissue in breasts and enlarge it naturally whereas the creams enlarge, firm, and reduce the appearance of stretch marks. The topical cream offers more benefits than the pill alone. Both claim to use all-natural herbs (Associated Press Online 2002; Guitierrez 2001; Milwaukee Journal Sentinel 2002; Minis 2002; PR Newswire 2002; Pravin 2002).

If taking pills or rubbing cream on the breasts is not to the liking of the consumer, there are numerous other solutions. Victoria's Secret was the first company to mass-market the Miracle Bra. From that, the Water Bra came into being—instead of having lifts that produce more cleavage, there is 'water' filled sacs on the underpinning of the support that give the breasts both a lift and a 'natural' look (Rana 2002). Finally, the most interesting product to me is the Brava Breast Enhancement and Shaping System. Brava consists of two plastic domes, a sports bra and a microprocessor-controlled device or "SmartBox", which creates a low vacuum that gently pulls the breast outward. Worn over 10 weeks, tissue expansion and swelling cause the breasts to enlarge. Around three or four weeks later, when swelling has subsided and the new tissue cells have stabilized, the breasts will have increased in volume by up to one cup size. Clinical trials in the United States have shown this product to be successful (Business Wire 2001; Litchfield 2002; Minis 2002).

In conclusion, countless institutions have emerged successfully on the market to combat obesity and enhance our physical appearance. It is amazing to me that our culture completely constructed this problem and it now has taken on a life of its own. The human body can be altered, shaped, and twisted into nearly any form imaginable; all the products on the market give the consumer the hope to do this within the framework of social acceptance. I believe that many citizens have forgotten, or are ignorant, to this construction. Many of them (as well as us) live in this reality and rarely have the opportunity for knowledge that allows us to see this matrix. When I see ads for these products on television, in magazines, and on the internet, I wonder what fool could possibly believe in the claims. Apparently millions do because this is a billion dollar industry that is only growing; the hope of physical perfection knows no monetary or safety value.

Frequency and Coding of Breast Enhancement Advertisements in Cosmopolitan and Seventeen Magazines: 1990-2000.

"By age 17, the traditionally socialized teenage girl will have learned, from many varied sources, that how she looks is more important than what she thinks, that her main goal in life is to find a man to take care of her financially, and that her place will be home with the kids and the cooking and the housework, while his place will be wherever he wants it to be" (Peirce 1990:491). I have observed this idea reproducing itself numerous times in my life. Look around! Look at women and observe how much make-up they put on. Look at how much time they obviously spend to fix their hair, and look at the calculated and precise manner in which most dress. I had two girlfriends in college who were willing to follow me wherever I went with the military at the expense of their aspirations after graduation. When I applied to law school, women came from everywhere, and many treated me in much higher regard after learning that I had been accepted to law school. Essentially, we reproduce the above quote through our assimilation and gender-role assignment processes and we can observe examples of such in our daily lives.

The idea of being attractive to the opposite sex begins when children enter adolescence. Boys and girls are both taught the ways in which the opposite sex will find them attractive. Boys are taught, through the media, that there is an ideal type of figure that a woman should have in order to be considered, attractive and girls aspire to become this image in order to gain attention from the boys. Thus, the media both teaches and scorns; it teaches by producing ideal types for both sexes to accept, yet scorns in that when a female does not fit the ideal type she is deemed "inadequate" by both boys and popular culture. "In fact, the American emphasis on female beauty becomes central to a teenage girl's life; it is the pretty girl and not the bright girl who is the most popular" (Romer 1981:56-57).

According to Peirce on the above basis, it is thus concluded that girl's achievement is directed towards winning social approval and other extrinsic rewards (Peirce 1990:495).

Another characteristic of female adolescence is the high regard that girls hold their boyfriends. Romer states that teenage girls tend to become very dependent on their boyfriends, and "they are frequently told that boyfriends are more important than grades and that good grades will not lead to popularity with the boys" (Romer 1981:56, 67). Thus, the definition of female success is based on attaining a desirable social status (through boyfriends), attractiveness to boys (understanding and conformity to such comes from the media), and marrying the right man (the first two dynamics combined). Upon review of literature and coming to such conclusions, I have decided to research the way in which the media conveys the definition of success to women through advertising because I believe that advertising is the root of the definition of success that women hold steadfast.

The basis of advertising towards females is to make them feel bad or guilty about not having a certain product. The product will do many things for the women—increase her attractiveness, boost her self-confidence, or possibly improve her quality of life. Essentially, her self-esteem and confidence are being attacked. This basis of advertising results in the self-esteem of the consumer dropping due to lack of access to the product. In a study by Polce-Lynch et. al. conducted, body image acted as a "filter" between media influence and self-esteem for girls, thus suggesting "the relationship between self-esteem and media may be more embedded in physical appearances for adolescent girls than for boys" (Polce-Lynch et. al.1991:240). They researched this very correlation to find that "...the influence of media played a unique role for girls in that media messages were associated with body image, which in turn was negatively associated with self-esteem" (Polce-Lynch et. al. 1991:239). Polce-Lynch et. al. furthered with defining which age group females were most likely to be impacted by advertising. They found that younger girls (being early to mid-adolescence) were most affected. "Cultural gender images, as communicated through television, movies, and advertisements, appear to be linked to the way these adolescences evaluated their physical appearances and themselves" (Polce-Lynch et. al. 1991:239). They concluded that body image continues to be associated with girl's self-esteem.

I want to explore the advertising aimed at adolescent girls and compare it to the advertising aimed at women. To do this, I have selected two magazines to use. Both magazines are the top two most popular women's glamour and fashion magazines and both are directed at a different audience. The first, *Seventeen*, has a large circulation of about 2.8 million as of 1997 (MPA Resources), has been in print since 1944, and is targeting girls thirteen to seventeen years of age (Peirce 1990:496). Peirce writes, "According to *Writer's Market 1989*, the magazine is geared toward young women concerned with the development of their own lives and the problems of the world around them" (Peirce 1990:496). She had a conversation with the managing editor the same year who told her "while the magazine is primarily fashion and beauty, their editorial purpose is to inform, entertain, and give teenage girls all the information they need to make sound choices in their lives. The fashion and beauty sections, she said, are to make the girls feel good about themselves" (Peirce1990:496-497). The second magazine is *Cosmopolitan,* published since 1952, marketing to women ages eighteen and up (although younger women do read it), and with an average circulation of 2.7 million as of 1998 (MPA Resources). *Cosmopolitan* picks up the audience that *Seventeen* graduates from high school, therefore looking at both will give me an idea of how the definition of success for a women is taught and reaffirmed through the transfer to adulthood.

I am going to summarize my study of *Cosmopolitan* first. I studied each issue for the past year (November 2000-November 2001) and looked for two types of advertisements: ads that were marketing weight-loss products and ads marketing breast enlargement procedures/products. Both types of ads used three dimensions for advertisement. First, the ads stated the scientific reasoning for the augmentation (often confusing). Second, the ads contained phrases to convince the consumer she would gain self-confidence from the product and third, the ads contained phrases hinting or directly stating that the consumer would be more desirable to the opposite sex by using the product. Thus, I have decided on two recording units. The first is going to be **references** to being better/more attractive to men or the current man in the consumers life. This also includes references that portray being inadequate because of not having used the product yet. Second, **phraseology** that states the consumer will feel better about herself for using the product (gained self-confidence). This also includes references that the user does not have self-confidence because they have not used the product yet. The intensity for both recording units is high due to the number of topics devoted to appearance; physical stature and breast size are base focuses. For example, when Peirce did a content analysis study of *Seventeen* magazine for the years 1961, 1972, and 1985, she calculated that appearance makes up 50% of the editorial content and that male-female relations takes up 7.0 and 6.5% of topic selection for the years 1961 and 1985, respectively (Peirce 1990: 498). One brief glance at *Cosmopolitan* will assure the reader that body image and male-female relations take up almost (at a rough estimate) 75% of magazine content. I am going to use frequency to measure the recording units.

Cosmopolitan had 64 advertisements marketing breast enlargement and 52 advertisements for weight loss. I also noticed that two of the same ads were never placed next to each other in the magazine; I would see a weight loss ad, then a breast enlargement ad, then a weight loss ad, and so forth. Using the definition of the first recording unit when studying the breast enlargement ads, I observed 36 references. Some examples are "People noticed, especially my husband" (Isis), "increase in actual cup size that everyone could see [obviously referring to men]" (Souage), and "women much less attractive than myself got more attention from men—just because they had fake breasts!" [Inferring gaining attention from having larger breasts than the narrator] (Full & Firm). Using the second recording unit for breast enlargement ads, I counted 40 phraseologies such as "I found it hard to look in the bathroom mirror naked" [the product will allow you to not do this] (Full & Firm) and "improve confidence" (in nearly *every* advertisement). The first and the second were combined in 8 cases, one being "It has been said a woman's bustline is her sexiest accessory. Improve your self confidence, make clothes fit better, and watch heads turn" (Full & Firm).

When using the first recording unit for weight loss ads, I observed 20 references with one being as direct as "It is a known fact—men are automatically drawn to a women with a lean, muscular body" (Liquatherm) and "...husband no longer interested in me at night" [using this product **will** regain his interest] (Geneva Bio-Science). When applying the second recording unit, I noted only 28 phraseologies such as "attain a slimmer, sexier body" (Herbal Body Wrap). In 8 advertisements (obviously repeat), the information given was strictly scientific and no recording unit could be applied.

I was surprised when I attempted to apply the two recording units to *Seventeen* magazine; they did not apply. I only saw one ad for breast enlargement (Bloussant) and it was small, without any references or phraseologies to record for, and relatively not eye-catching. I did not observe any verbally direct advertising as blatant as that in *Cosmopolitan* magazine. What I did observe were advertisements of summer camps were girls could go to lose weight. These ads intensified in frequency the months precluding the school summer break (January-May). The only reoccurring ideological phrase of the advertisements was that of losing weight and keeping it off. I studied all issues for the year of 2000 and that of 1980. In the 2000 issues, I counted 16 ads for summer weight loss camps from the months January to June and 1 ad for weight loss camps from July to December (the ad was in the July issue). What I did find, however, were advertisements

for modeling agencies/programs. 52 advertisements appeared throughout the
year with about 5 each month. Oddly enough, the issues spanning the 1980 year
had nearly the same numbers of 20 ads for weight loss camps (slightly higher) and
50 advertisements for modeling agencies/programs. As with 2000, the weight loss
camps were at their advertisement peak in the months of January to June.

Seventeen magazine was hard to decipher. Even though there were not blatant
verbal references to record for, the same ideology existed. For example, all of the
modeling agency/program advertisements showed a busty, thin teenage girl. *Seventeen* magazine employs the same ideology as *Cosmopolitan* magazine, but
directed at a younger audience. Both have "quizzes" related to male-female relations. Both use the theme of "getting the best boy/man" with a busty, thin
women directly under or around the title of the article. I now argue that advertising uses imaging to give an ideal type to teenage girls, directly market them when
they are of consensual age (by graduating to *Cosmopolitan)*, and finalizing it when
they have the financial resources to purchase the products.

I realize this study is grossly incomplete. To further this, I would like to go
into deeper content analysis by assigning recording units to the articles. After
studying so many magazines, I observed direct parallels between article content in
both magazines orbiting around the central theme of impressing and ultimately
capturing "a man" in the reader's life. Peirce concluded her study of *Seventeen*
magazine by stating, "A teenage girl, then, should be concerned with her appearance, with finding a man to take care of her, and with learning to take care of a
house…according to the managing editor, giving them what they want is not the
purpose of the publication. Giving them the information they need in their lives
is" (Peirce 1990:499). Once again, who determines what teenage girls need in
their lives?

The Marijuana Tax Act

The Marijuana Tax Act is a bill that was passed in 1937 by the federal government concerning the selling, cultivating, and bartering of cannabis. It required that the seller, purchaser and cultivator of any derivative of the cannabis plant to buy a stamp from the government. The stamp cost a lot of money and the tax that accompanied made it near impossible economically for anyone to purchase or cultivate hemp. Laws against marijuana smoking were left to the preference of individual states. Each state adopted such laws before the passage of the Marijuana Tax Act, although loosely enforced them until the mid 1930's. How were the states laws against marijuana smoking affected by the Marijuana Tax Act? What is the Marijuana Tax Act and how was it enacted into a law? Why was marijuana smoking such a prominent issue in the 1930's, or as sociologists ponder, why now?

Sociology of law is the study of how society structures itself in accordance to law. Law is always treated as a dependent variable because laws are culture and time specific. There are no universal rights or wrongs; members of societies create laws dependent on the opinion of the majority of the members within that society. Laws are a reflection of the members of a society because they reflect the values and norms held by such. Thus, one could argue that the heavily taxation of hemp and making marijuana smoking illegal reflects the value that Americans did not want the tax-free bartering and selling of hemp nor recreational marijuana smoking accepted any longer. I am arguing this contention because after review and study of reasons for prohibiting recreational marijuana use and further taxing its use for industrial purposes, I firmly believe that it was a matter of a few elite individuals using a propaganda campaign to scare the American people into believing that hemp and its derivatives are evil in order to protect their economic interests.

Hemp (the plant that marijuana is derived from) has been a most useful plant to man for thousands of years. From it is produced durable fiber which can be woven into anything; its centers, or "hurds", make excellent paper and its seeds are full of protein that make great lubrication when pressed. Extracts from its leaves have provided a wide range of medicines and tonics (Herer 1998).

Hemp has also been used profusely in the history of the United States. George Washington and Thomas Jefferson, our beloved forefathers, grew hemp. Our first American flag was sown on hemp cloth. The first and second drafts of the Declaration of Independence were written on paper made from Dutch hemp, and when the pioneers went west they covered their wagons with hemp cloths. Mary Todd (Abraham Lincoln's wife) came from the richest hemp growing family in Kentucky (Herer 1998).

After the Civil War, hemp cloth production in the United States greatly decreased because it became too expensive without slave labor. Cotton ginned by machines was cheaper. Even though hemp had a high production cost, it still remained the second most popular cloth in America. Hemp rope was the mainstay of the Navy. Two thousand tons of hempseed were sold annually as birdfeed. Virtually all good paints and varnishes were made from hemp-seed oil (Herer 1998). Hemp's by-products remained popular until the Marijuana Tax Act was passed in 1937. What happened? How could a plant with so many uses and with such a long, popular history in our country be demonized?

Before I begin to discuss how the Marijuana Tax Act passed and recreational marijuana smoking made illegal, we must first look at the historical context in which all of the controversy arose. Once again law, as a dependent variable, is relative to the time and culture in which it is serving. We must understand what was happening socially in the 1920's and 1930's that led to such an enormous scare against hemp and marijuana smoking.

The Great Depression swallowed our country in 1929. It was a time of economic crisis; money and jobs were scarce. The very security and comfort of the lives of American citizens was being challenged, and no end to the problem seemed to be in sight.

Mexicans began immigrating, in great numbers, to the south and southwest of our country in the mid 1920's. They primarily worked in agriculture and provided a cheap source of labor for farms and orchards. When the Great Depression struck, many Mexicans migrated north to the central plain states looking for work. They were already being paid a substandard wage and were paid less during the Depression. Americans thought that Mexicans were taking their place in the labor force. They became a scapegoat for the lack of employment through a commonly held belief that they were taking all the jobs. People panicked because of the unstable times. Citizens, also afraid of mixing with an "inferior race", formed groups such as "Allied Patriotic Societies", "Key Men in America", or the group that unified many of these associations, "American Coalition" (Musto 1973).

Mexicans smoked marijuana for recreational purposes and brought this habit with them when they immigrated and further migrated. They were also labeled as violent individuals who would use knives in fights, and such a label helped create a menacing tie between marijuana usage and consequences thereof. This anti-Mexican sentiment in association with marijuana smoking was the genesis of the marijuana scare that enveloped our country in the mid 1930's (Himmelstein 1983).

Himmelstein argues a theory he calls, "social locus". This theory contends that there is "a relationship between the moral and legal status of a particular kind of drug use and the social position of the groups identified as the primary or typical users; the lower the social position of the users, the more likely that use will be regarded as deviant, disreputable, and wrong. As the social location of use changes, so does its moral status" (Himmelstein 1983: 16). As such, when smoking marijuana was associated with Mexicans who as a group were stereotyped as violent and already occupied a low social position, the moral and legal status of marijuana also diminished.

Why were the Mexicans singled out as a minority and stereotyped? Along with the perceived notion in the 1930's that Mexicans were taking all the agriculture jobs in the Midwest and South, Gusfield postulates a theory that deals with drugs and drug controls as symbolic encounters in wider social conflicts. During times of great social conflict or stress (the Depression), the drug use of a socially subordinate or insurgent group may become a symbol of the threat that the group poses to the dominant social order. "Legislation against the drug in association may be a way of reasserting the legitimacy of the existing social hierarchy and the hegemony of dominant social groups by symbolically condemning those groups which threaten that hierarchy and hegemony." (Himmelstein 1983: 17). Thus, the immediate enforcement of already existing laws against the recreational use of marijuana could have been a way to re-establish the subordination of Mexicans and reaffirm the status (law making and majority) of the white dominant group (Himmelstein 1983).

Precedent had been set concerning other substances that were used for recreational pleasure. The Prohibition Act in 1920 made it illegal to manufacture or sell "intoxicating liquors" (though ended in 1933). The Harrison Act, passed in 1914, federally required individuals to register if they were dealing with narcotic drugs (both medically and personally). Precedents had been set against substances people used for pleasure, and legislating a law whose ultimate goal would be to ban marijuana (by attacking hemp) appeared to be easier and only a matter of time (Heiligman 1992).

How did the Federal Government legitimize the prohibition of alcohol and opium? The following "values" were used as a justification:

1. Protestant Ethic—individuals should exercise complete responsibility for what he or she does and what happens to him or her; a person should never do anything that might result in the loss of self-control. Alcohol and opiates cause loss of self-control; therefore, they are evil.

2. Disapproval of Action Based Solely to Achieve Status of Ecstasy—because of our cultural emphasis on pragmatism and utilitarianism, citizens feel uneasy and ambivalent about ecstatic experiences of any kind.

3. Humanitarianism—reformers believed that people "enslaved" by the use of alcohol and opium would benefit from laws making it impossible for them to give in to their weaknesses (Becker 1976).

These same values were used when attempting to legitimize the Marijuana Tax Act because people smoked marijuana for pleasure.

A depression hit the economy of the United States and disenfranchised the whole country, marijuana smoking had been tied to a minority group, and precedent had been set by the government concerning its right to judge the effects of recreational substances and when they could and could not be used. How did the government become involved with marijuana smoking laws and what gave them the legitimate right to do such?

All members in the society that accept what actions the enforcers take legitimize government and law enforcement bodies, according to the Structural-Functionalist theory of Emile Durkheim. Since people elect to have a law enforcement body support the will of the majority, accepting those laws enacted (from strong reactions towards a particular behavior) legitimizes the law itself and conversely reflects the collective conscious of a society. Citizens in the South and Midwest were complaining to local law enforcement, who in turn complained to state law enforcement, who finally complained to federal law enforcement and government about marijuana smoking and its violent effects. Oddly enough, the complaints did not occur on a grand scale until after the Depression and the migration of Mexican workers. Regardless, the complaints began to bring more attention to the issue because there was now a public sentiment against marijuana smoking. This enlisted the aid of local, state, and federal law enforcement individuals to bring attention (and later legislation) to the issue.

The government officials and supporters who enacted legislation against hemp and marijuana smoking were "moral entrepreneurs". Becker urges us to pay attention to those social groups and organizations who took the initiative to procure a particular drug law as well as how and why they did so. Moral rules, as Becker reminds us, are not automatically created and enforced. "Rule creation and enforcement require 'moral enterprise', the specific effort by a formally constituted agent to transform established social values into specific rules and then see to it that these rules are applied. Such an agent is a "moral entrepreneur" (Himmelstein 1983: 15). Becker states that to procure a new moral rule, the moral entrepreneur must go through a characteristic process of publicizing the area of wrongdoing, enlisting organizational support, and cultivating public opinion. Further in this paper, when we observe how a propaganda campaign was started to rally public support, we see that the latter theory in action. What government agencies and individuals became the moral entrepreneurs against hemp and marijuana smoking?

The Federal Bureau of Narcotics was created on August 12, 1930. It was created as independent from the Treasury Department and Harry J. Anslinger was appointed the first commissioner under president Herbert Hoover. Harry J. Anslinger is the moral entrepreneur who is single-handedly responsible for the passage of the Marijuana Tax Act in 1937. Anslinger had stiff policies that he applied in dealing with narcotics and believed that the only way to enforce drug laws was to have stiff penalties (this philosophy characterized the Federal Bureau of Narcotics attitude for years to come). The Federal Bureau of Narcotics joined the fight supporting drug legislation because Congress re-examined all federal expenditures in the first years of the Depression and cut the Federal Bureau of Narcotics payroll by 200,000 dollars. Anslinger was fearful that the Bureau would be totally ousted, so he realized that he had to give a reason or provide some kind of mission to legitimize the Federal Bureau of Narcotics and it's existence. "Anslinger had to prove that there was a new drug menace threatening the country, one that required immediate federal attention, one that the Bureau of Narcotics could deal with only if it's hands weren't tied" (Abel 1980: 240). Anslinger had to prove such reality and created a menace. He realized the force of public opinion, and used it to begin a propaganda campaign that would ultimately result in the Marijuana Tax Act (Abel 1980).

"Harry J. Anslinger set about to promote the notion that the marijuana smoker was a serious threat and was responsible for an increasing number of crimes, particularly crimes of violence including murder and rape" (Salmon 1972: 24). Anslinger realized, very ingeniously, that he could play on the Mexican stereotype to exploit the largeness of the situation. He wanted to conclusively link marijuana smoking to the Mexican minority. He had great political power to do so because he raised the support of both Republicans and Democrats, the Women's Christian Temperance Union, and many churches. Because the Federal Bureau of Narcotics also controlled the licenses for the importation of opiates, Anslinger also received support from the drug companies. While exploiting these fears and cultivating special interest groups, he also utilized the demographic changes in the "addict" population (including a growing number of Mexicans) (Galliher, Keys, Elsner 1998).

Harry Anslinger was also a savvy bureaucrat during the Great Depression who excelled at protecting the Federal Bureau of Narcotics from budget cuts by locating new legislative mandates. Anslinger, above all, was a government operative with vast experience in the intelligence community who, through political harassment, adeptly controlled the flow of information on drug addiction. Anslinger was a moral entrepreneur as well as a moral enforcer. He used his position, prestige, and power in the Federal Bureau of Narcotics to define his position on the supposed drug problem, mobilize legislative initiatives, and to implement law enforcement plans of action. This is all essential in creating a social problem, which Anslinger did (Galliher, Keys, Elsner 1998).

"In fact, the Bureau (FBN) had no obvious or natural interest in procuring national marijuana controls. To be sure, it was a survival-conscious bureaucracy and its leaders were moralists to the core, but neither fact pre-disposed it to seek control over marijuana, or for that matter, over barbiturates and amphetamines" (Himmelstein 1983: 138-39). The "war" against hemp and marijuana smoking was now afoot in order to give the Federal Bureau of Narcotics a mission, which in turn legitimized its existence and kept it from receiving further budget cuts. An enemy was created. The Marijuana Tax Act was born out of legislation to control marijuana smoking. What was the Marijuana Tax Act? How did Anslinger organize a propaganda campaign to gain support from the American people? Did Anslinger work in his own self-interest (did Anslinger directly benefit in any way from pushing such an agenda)?

The Federal Bureau of Narcotics left the acceptance and enforcement of recreational marijuana smoking strictly to individual state preference. It was the choice of the state to include marijuana in their State Uniform Narcotic Act. By 1930, sixteen states had passed laws prohibiting smoking marijuana for recreational use. These laws were loosely enforced, and states had little to no complaints with linking ill activity to marijuana smoking In 1931, thirteen more states followed suit, making a total of twenty-nine. This exemplifies that marijuana smoking was already a local issue and it shows how the Federal Bureau of Narcotics became aware of the "problem" (Himmelstein 1983). In 1932, the Federal Bureau of Narcotics began working directly with the National Conference of Commissioners on Uniform State Laws in developing uniform laws concerning narcotics, stressing the need to control marijuana (Becker 1976). This is when Harry Anslinger began his campaign against marijuana smoking.

The issue remained stagnant and of little concern to local law enforcement and even the Federal Bureau of Narcotics. The complaints were minimal and Anslinger had no case against marijuana or hemp. Finally, in 1934, a law was passed that gave Anslinger the idea on how to completely ban hemp. In the effort to reduce the number of sub-machine guns being bought and sold by gangsters, Congress decreed that such firearms could not be transferred without a tax (and that tax was very hefty). This was called the Firearm Transfer Tax. Anslinger realized that if he could get the same legislation passed for hemp (by heavily taxing the transfer and cultivation of it), he could completely eliminate it from the market for production and sale. From such, stricter enforcement of marijuana smoking laws would ensue. Farmers could not afford heavy taxes on major commodities, and hemp was a major commodity for all farmers that cultivated it. Even though Anslinger was somewhat skeptical about the legitimacy or such legislation passing, it provided a framework for him as well as a legal precedent to cite (Musto 1973).

Anslinger and the Federal Bureau of Narcotics continued to work on an anti-marijuana campaign. Support for such a law was so little that only three of the twelve states that adopted the State Uniform Narcotic Act in 1935 included recreational marijuana smoking as a crime. Anslinger realized that he needed to rally support quickly; the Federal Bureau of Narcotics had little or no mission and was having a very difficult time pushing the anti-marijuana agenda. They needed to arouse public concern about marijuana smoking. He needed to convince citizens that marijuana smoking was responsible for all social problems (Helmer 1975).

Anslinger began supplying propaganda to community service clubs and popular press concerning alleged atrocities committed by those under the influence of marijuana. He flooded the press with stories to get the attention of the average citizen. The following are excerpts from articles that Anslinger wrote himself and that appeared nine times in popular magazines between 1936-1937:

> "The sprawled body of a young girl lay crushed on the sidewalk the other day after a plunge from the fifth story of a Chicago apartment house. Everyone called it suicide, but it was actually murder. The killer was a narcotic used in

the form of a cigarette comparatively new to the United States and as dangerous as a coiled rattlesnake" (Anslinger and Cooper 1937: 19).

This article appeared five times in popular magazines from 1936-1937:

> "An entire family was murdered by a youthful [marijuana] addict in Florida. When the officers arrived at the house they found the youth staggering about in human slaughter-house. With an axe he had killed his father, mother, two brothers, and a sister. He seemed to be in a daze...he had no recollection of having committed the multiple crimes. The officers knew him ordinarily as a sane, rather quiet young man; now he was pitifully crazed. They sought the reason. The boy said that he had been in the habit of smoking something which the youthful friends called "muggles", a childish name for marijuana" (Anslinger and Cooper 1937: 150).

The above was a typical way for the Federal Bureau of Narcotics to describe the drug, it's influences, it's identification, and it's "evil" effects (Abel 1980).

Marijuana smoking laws were the business of the states and federal intervention would be unjustifiable. In order to obtain federal intervention, Anslinger's attention turned toward more deviant ways of getting what he wanted. He calculated that if the United States became part of an international drug treaty that a federal law would have to be passed despite opposition on constitutional grounds to any law restricting cannabis on the basis of current federal tax or interstate laws. Anslinger cited the Migratory Bird Act, which was upheld to be constitutional by the Supreme Court, to combat the opposition above. The Act was declared constitutional even though it overstepped state police powers due to the fact that it was an international treaty with Canada and Mexico. Therefore, he could not receive opposition when he decided to go to Geneva in June of 1936 to attend the conference for the "Suppression of Illicit Traffic in Dangerous Drugs" and urge other countries to adopt controls in trafficking cannabis. If other countries adopted such controls along with the United States, then a federal law would have to be passed and the individual states would be forced to comply. The other countries did not agree with him; they argued that his medical evidence was not valid because it did not study the total effects of marijuana on the human body (Musto 1973). Defeated internationally, Anslinger returned home to further fight for federal legislation.

Anslinger continued to successfully flood the press with propaganda and turn the sentiment of citizens against marijuana smoking. The Federal Bureau of Narcotics urged the National Conference of Commissioners on Uniform Narcotic

State Laws in 1936 that federal intervention may be necessary because the problem was getting "out of control". They wanted to work with them in order to "educate" people on the effects of marijuana smoking (Becker 1976). Anslinger felt that he finally had enough public support to proceed to the next level. In January of 1937, he held a conference in the Treasury Building. His goal was to create a final legislation to submit to Congress. When creating the evidence to support their cause, they fabricated their medical reports and did not hear any evidence unless it directly agreed with their agenda (Musto 1973). The finalized bill contained the following information:

1.   Handlers of cannabis had to register and had to pay a special "occupational tax".

2.   Written forms had to be submitted and filed for every transaction involving cannabis, and payment of a transfer tax of one dollar per ounce had to be paid each time the drug was delivered to an authorized recipient (a HUGE tax at that time) (Abel 1980).

The Firearms Transfer Tax was finally declared constitutional in April of 1937. This set the perfect precedent for the Federal Bureau of Narcotics and Anslinger to proceed. One month later, Anslinger and the Treasury Department presented the bill before the House Ways and Means Committee. What ensued was a tragedy to the American legal system (Musto 1973).

Anslinger knew that in order to convince the House to pass the bill they would have to focus on the "ill effects" of marijuana smoking and not the bill itself (which only entailed cannabis handling). There were no practical reasons for the government to regulate hemp, and by demonstrating that a derivative of the plant caused atrocities would aid in the passage of the bill. Anslinger knew that once the government regulated trade and production, they could assure that production and trade disappeared.

The violence claim was Anslinger's main angle and contention that dominated the Congressional Hearings. The Federal Bureau of Narcotics stressed that marijuana smoking stimulated violent behavior by dissolving moral restraints, by destroying the ability to judge from right and wrong, by stimulating grandiose fantasies, and by making the user highly suggestible. Violence was also the central theme of the three articles and two of the four letters submitted as exhibits to the Committee (Himmelstein 1983).

They also knew that Congress would not believe the "hype" they had released to the newspapers and magazines without sufficient medical backing. Strangely, the Federal Bureau of Narcotics main medical witness *was* Harry Anslinger. Not only that, but they had a pharmacologist named James Munch testify (whose research concerning the effects of marijuana was focused on dogs). He had given them marijuana to eat to observe if it altered their personalities. When asked about the altering of their personalities, he stated, "Yes, as far as I can tell, not being a dog psychologist" (Abel 1980: 244). This was actually allowed as testimony before the House Ways and Means Committee!

The American Medical Association was contacted to appear at the hearing. They sent spokesperson Dr. William Woodard. Dr. Woodard was appalled at the evidence Anslinger produced before the House being that Anslinger was not a doctor and had no legitimate evidence to support his claims concerning the effects of marijuana. Dr. Woodard had not prepared evidence to bring the House because the American Medical Association had no idea that the effects of marijuana smoking were being "researched", let alone for the past two years. When Dr. Woodard gave testimony, he stated before the House that Anslinger's evidence was completely fabricated; the American Medical Association had no idea that a bill was being created, and that they had only been notified one month in advance before appearing. Dr. Woodard asked for an extension and six months to gather evidence and fully evaluate Anslinger's claims. He was denied. Dr. Woodard and the American Medical Association were particularly upset with this because the Harrison Act led to the annoyance and harassment of physicians. Many doctors felt that this infringed on their professional right to treat patients how they saw fit. Marijuana was widely used and recognized for its medicinal effects. Dr. Woodard and the American Medical Association knew they if this bill passed, they would no longer be allowed to treat patients with such medicines as they see fit (Abel 1980).

Why did the House Ways and Means Committee ignore the pleas and professional opinion of Dr. Woodard? The American Medical Association had recently successfully blocked health insurance from being included in the Social Security Act, therefore leaving the House with a very sour sentiment towards them (Abel 1980). They were in no mood to hear the American Medical Association, nor Dr. Woodard.

"After hearings, the bill went to the House of Representatives. Before the bill was voted on, a short exchange took place showing that Congress was not even aware of what the drug marijuana was (though the bill entailed the taxation of hemp), even though they were being asked to outlaw its use!

<u>Mr. Snell</u>: What is the bill?

<u>Mr. Rayburn</u>: It has something to do with something that is called marijuana. I believe that it is a narcotic of some kind" (Abel 1980: 247).

Finally, the House passed the bill and it was shortly sent back to the Senate. The Senate amended it and sent it back to the House, which passed it with no roll call or debate. The Marijuana Tax Act was passed and signed by President Roosevelt on August 2, 1937. It went into effect October 1, 1937. The passing only merited three lines of discussion in the New York Times the day it was signed (Abel 1980).

The Marijuana Tax Act did not make hemp or marijuana illegal; it simply meant that for a person to cultivate and market hemp, one would have to purchase a "stamp" and pay taxes, both cultivator (now regulated by the government) and the purchaser. These taxes were very high and no one (especially farmers) could afford it. It made hemp products economically ridiculous to pay for. It cost so much to purchase hemp by-products that no profit would be made once they sold (if at all because of the extraordinary high price due to taxation) on the market.

Congress declared the possession of cannabis (or any derivative thereof) without a stamp to be a felony, and there were practically no stamps to be bought (Musto 2000). The federal government involved itself with marijuana smoking by making a possession law. This allowed the states to retain their individual laws concerning marijuana smoking. The states felt that they had retained their autonomy and the Federal Bureau of Narcotics became involved nationally, thus pacifying all parties involved.

I read the latter happenings, from the beginning of the Federal Bureau of Narcotics to the ridiculousness of the trial, and still have questions. It appears there had to be *some* other ulterior motive for Anslinger to be a moral entrepreneur. I understand that Anslinger used his political clout to create an enemy and thus created a mission for the Federal Bureau of Narcotics, but it perhaps seems that he had another reason for attacking hemp so profusely without retreating until he achieved his objective. The following is a very interesting conspiracy theory, which provides a motive that Anslinger appeared to have through association with certain individuals.

Hemp, for all practical purposes, was outlawed just as a new technology would have made hemp paper much cheaper than wood-pulp paper. Hemp fiber had to be separated from the stalk by hand. The cost of labor made this method uncompetitive. The year that hemp was taxed (1937), a machine was invented named the *decorticator*. It could process as much as three tons of hemp an hour and could produce higher quality fibers with a lot less fiber than wood-based pulp.

Some scientists predicated that hemp would have been able to undercut the competition overnight. *Popular Mechanics* predicted that hemp would become the United States first billion-dollar crop. The magazine pointed out that 10,000 acres of hemp would produce as much paper as 40,000 acres of forestland (Herer 1998). "Hearst, the du Ponts, and other industrial barons and financiers knew that the machinery to cut, bale, decorticate (separate fiber from the stalk) and process hemp into paper was becoming available in the mid-1930's" (Herer 1998: 41).

William Randolph Hearst was a prominent magazine owner and businessman from the early to mid 1900's. As exemplification of his empire, Hearst built a castle on a 240,000-acre ranch at San Simeon, California in the 1920's. At his peak he owned twenty-eight major newspapers and eighteen magazines, along with several radio stations and movie companies. According to Herer, Hearst slanted the news in his papers to protect his wood pulp investments. Hearst's newspaper chain led a campaign to have hemp outlawed. He falsified stories and made claims as outrageous as Anslinger's. Herer furthers that Hearst was responsible for popularizing the term, "marijuana". The first step in creating hysteria, for Hearst, was to introduce a foreign word that would scare people; thus, he coined the Spanish word "marijuana" (Herer 1998).

The Du Pont Company also had a large part in such a conspiracy. They had been a major manufacturer of textiles and gunpowder from the mid 1800's through the Second World War. They had an economic interest in the wood pulp industry as well. At this time, they were in the process of patenting a new sulfuric acid process for producing wood pulp paper. According to the company's *own* record, nearly eighty percent of all Du Pont's railroad car loadings for the next fifty years would contain wood pulp products. Even more of a reason for Du Pont to be concerned would be their changing business and manufacturing practices after World War One. They poured millions of dollars in developing synthetic fibers such as rayon and nylon during the peacetime following the war predicting that such products would be more profitable in the long run. Hemp can be woven into rope and clothing providing the strongest natural fiber in the world. In 1935, Du Pont developed nylon that was a substitute for hemp rope. In 1939, they developed rayon, which was a direct competitor against hemp cloth. To make things deeper, Congress and the Treasury Department were promised through testimony given by Du Pont that hemp seed oil could be replaced with synthetic petrochemical oil produced by Du Pont. The millions spent on these products as well as the hundreds of millions expected from profit could have been wiped out if the newly affordable hemp products were allowed on the market. Du Pont worked with Hearst to eliminate hemp (Herer 1998).

How was Harry Anslinger involved? He was Du Pont's "point man". Andrew Mellon, who had appointed Anslinger as commissioner of the Federal Bureau of Narcotics under Herbert Hoover, was also chairman of the Mellon Bank, which was Du Pont's main financial backer. Anslinger just also happened to be married to Mellon's niece (Herer 1998). Could this all be a happenstance? I do not believe so. I believe that the evidence provided above proves that Anslinger had an ulterior motive other than creating a mission for the Federal Bureau of Narcotics.

The Marijuana Tax Act had a long history before its passage. The Harrison Act was the first federal ruling concerning the trafficking of narcotics. The Prohibition Act made it illegal to produce or serve alcohol. These two acts provided framework for the precedent of making further rulings on conscious-altering substances. The Great Depression came in 1929, redefining the normative order daily as the economy collapsed and could not recuperate. The migration of Mexicans to the Midwest and providing competition for unemployed citizens created hatred and thus designated the Mexican migrant worker as a scapegoat. Their practice of recreational marijuana smoking tied their behavior and minority status to an activity that had been previously accepted. Harry Anslinger and the Federal Bureau of Narcotics were receiving major budget cutbacks due to the Great Depression and needed to create a mission for them to legitimize their existence. Observing a minor public sentiment against marijuana smoking in the Midwest and Western states along with the few complaints of law enforcement officials, Anslinger realized that he could turn the emotions of disenfranchised citizens of the United States against marijuana, thus creating a mission for the Federal Bureau of Narcotics by becoming federally involved. Combined with his connection to millions of dollars Du Pont and Hearst stood to loose, he used the Firearms Tax Act and the Migratory Bird Act as frameworks for creating the Marijuana Tax Act. Harry Anslinger launched a campaign to scare the American people and rallied public support for his bill. He abused his political clout and connections to ultimately have the Marijuana Tax Act passed in 1937, forever changing the public view and norms concerning hemp and recreational marijuana smoking. The true question is if Anslinger and the Federal Bureau of Narcotics were so adamant about fixing the supposed marijuana smoking "problem", why did they not enact legislation on the federal level concerning the issue? In other words, why would Anslinger push to pass a hemp law verses a marijuana smoking law if marijuana smoking and its direct "ill effects" were the concern?

The horror stories (apparently resulting from smoking) were the focal point to rally public support for Anslinger's real issue of protecting his kin's economic interest by crippling the hemp threat. However, I do think that it was genius to achieve the goal of outlawing marijuana and eradicate the economic threat of hemp all in one bill.

Law is treated as a dependent variable because it changes from time to time and place to place. I do not believe, after my research, that the Marijuana Tax Act served much social purpose other than to flood the economy with new products (as replacements for existing hemp products) and demonize a minority group in our country. However, I do understand how Anslinger used the sentiment of the public and their emotions against them to achieve his goal. The American people were very vulnerable at that time and were looking for the government to pull them from the tragic Depression. Anslinger used this to his benefit.

After completing the research and writing this paper, I am infuriated. I realize that the anti-marijuana campaign that I have been assimilated to my entire life is nothing more than the result of a conspiracy by a few powerful men who wanted to protect their economic interests. I believe that the intentions of Anslinger were to protect his interest along with the individuals (Hearst and Du Pont) and not for the good of the country. I have strayed away from the usage of marijuana and labeled users as deviants due to my ignorance of the subject and the culture in which I was raised. I am slowly learning to question every facet of my normative order to understand the true meaning and reasoning surrounding public policies and issues. This research has opened my eyes to corruption, conspiracy, and the power that one calculating bureaucrat can have on a country in his time as well as years to come after his death.

The American people became adamantly against the recreational use of marijuana because of the propaganda that flooded the media. We accept things face value and truthful because most of us have no reason to question the underlined meaning behind many issues. The American people in the 1930's followed the trend created by Anslinger and did not question the sources or legitimacy of his information. They accepted it because if such stories were in their favorite magazines and the source is the commissioner of a government agency, then it *must* be true. I do not fault the citizens of the United States; they truly did not know any better at the time.

This research paper has made my cynical. My opinions about marijuana and other drugs that I came across in my research have changed forever. I find that I have more distrust now. I believe that once I asked "why now" in regards to as why the Marijuana Tax Act came into existence and passed. I have answered the question. I plan on making numerous copies of this paper and distributing it to all of my friends and family that are willing to read this. We all need to be aware of our government, its underline policies, and the context in which laws are made.

Conclusion

In conclusion, I believe that I have presented sufficient material to explain how the media has duped women into hating themselves. This is the psychological advertisement technique used to sell products to women, but the personal repercussions are not taken into account. I do not believe that the advertising agencies *intended* for women to engage in such practices as eating disorders and to have self-esteem issues; they are social consequences of internalized advertisement consumption.

The only way that women can be truly free is to understand the 'matrix' of advertising code set forth in this text. This understanding will lead to more educated decision making processes. Even though the conscious decision is made to pay attention to media outlets [thereby consuming the advertisements], purchase products, and engage in destructive personal behavior, the root of the decision is so far ingrained within women [through cultural assimilation] that the fundamental question of 'why' is not addressed. For clarification, I mean that women who engage in an act such as bulimia [social consequence/malady as an example] do not ask themselves why they are doing it; they simply have a conscious means to a given goal [lose weight, self-hate in a sadistic reification, ect.]. The 'why' is explained through the forces of advertising that I have accurately and historically traced.

Capitalism and the selling of products rests on the freedom of personal expression. We believe that we are expressing ourselves through the purchases that we make. Our cars, clothes, and houses define who we are as people. We are taught that our purchases are expressions of who we are as an individual. Every product marketed has a demographic or target audience. Why would it be so hard to believe that we are all reproducing the images of the media presentations of the lifestyle that we follow or believe in? Women are doing this by putting on make-up, wearing prescribed types of clothing, and purchasing based on the expressing their personal desires [or so they believe]. They conform to the presented sub-culture they wish to be associated with, and the advertisements targeting that sub-culture are based on guilt, fear, and inadequacy.

People do not like to entertain the ideas that I write about. They do not want to believe that their personal expression of self is nothing more than a marketing ploy aimed at making money. People do not like to have their belief system questioned because it usurps their reality. They do not want to entertain the idea that The Marijuana Tax Act was passed due to Anslinger's agenda and, moreover, that much of the information presented by the media about marijuana is false. Women do not want to believe that they have been taught to hate themselves in order to buy products that will supposedly make them feel better. Our culture deems each individual their own God and gives us the right to self-determination. Believing that someone or something else is the puppeteer of our decisions is an unmentionable and often unexplored topic.

I included the bonus chapter on The Marijuana Tax Act in order to demonstrate that a few people, with and agenda and power, can launch advertising and propaganda campaigns that can effectively change the reality we live in. Only a handful of people that are anti-marijuana could tell you any of the information that I explored—they know a few buzz words and phrases they grew up with and saw on television. Most cannot even tell you that much and many get angry when their beliefs are questioned. This is characteristic of most commonly-held beliefs. Take the war in Iraq for example—many people in our country [when Gallup polled], *although thoroughly disproved*, still believe that Iraq and Sadaam Hussein were linked with 9/11 and that President Bush invaded the country for Democracy. That is wrong. Film makers such as Michael Moore present a well thought-out and researched alternative opinion, but it is dismissed by the same people who would dismiss the writings in this text; entertaining such ideas forces them outside of their comfort zone and the ideas are met with anger and refute.

I urge everyone is society to think and question the world around them. Without thought and questions, we are nothing more than sheep to the slaughter. An obedient society allows those that do think, in powerful positions, to decide for the rest of us. Let us not forget that solutions are often invented before the problem exists and solutions are created by those with a political or financial agenda.

Bibliography

Abel, Ernest L. 1980. *Marihuana: The First Twelve Thousand Years*. New York, NY: Plenum Press.

Altheide, David L.1996. *Qualitative Media Analysis*. Newbury Park, CA: Sage.

Anslinger, Harry J. and C.R. Cooper. 1937. "Marihuana: Assassin of Youth." *American Magazine* July: 19-22.

Associated Press Online. 2002. "Company to Stop Selling Breast Cream, Pills." *Associated Press Online*. December 31. Washington Dateline. Retrieved on February 5, 2003 (http://web.lexis-nexis.com/universe/document?_m=b154940 ad7ae61b9623f12750faca685&_docnum=11&wchp=dGLbVlb-lSlAl&_md5= 1c12f9eaee0dfefae2d8683576fa44fa).

Bergerson, Sherry M. and Charlene Y. Senn. 1998. "Body Image and Sociocultural Norms." *Psychology of Women Quarterly* 22: 385-401.

Best, Joel (Ed). 1995. *Images of Issues: Typifying Contemporary Social Problems*. 2nd Edition. New York, NY: Aldine de Gruyter.

Bloom, Howard.1995. *The Lucifer Principle*. New York, NY: The Atlantic Monthly Press.

Bordo, Susan. 1993. "Hunger as Ideology." Pp. 99-114 in *The Consumer Society Reader* edited by Juliet B. Schor and Douglas B. Holt. New York, NY: The New Press.

------. 1993. *Unbearable Weight: Feminism, Western Culture, and The Body*. Berkley, CA: University of California Press.

------. 1990. "Material Girl: The Effacements of Postmodern Culture." *Michigan Quarterly Review* 29: 653-677.

Business Wire. 2001. Advancement in Non-Surgical Breast Enlargement Technology." *Business Wire.* May 23, Healthwire. Retrieved on February 24, 2003 (http://web.lexis-nexis.com/universe/document?_m=b154940ad7ae61b 9623f12750faca685&_docnum=3&wchp=dGLbVlb-lSlAl&_md5=3ff1b 208440ae5c4e48e238ccac5584f).

Campbell, Collin. 1991. "Consumption: The New Wave of Research in the Humanities and Social Sciences." Pp. 33-36 in *The Consumer Society* edited by Neva R. Goodwin, Frank Ackerman, and David Kiron. Covelo, CA: Island Press.

Courtney, Alice E. and Sarah Wernick Lockeretz. 1978. "A Woman's Place: An Analysis of Roles Portrayed by Women in Magazine Advertisements." *Journal of Marketing Research* 14: 92-95.

Davis, Kathy. 1995. *Reshaping the Female Body: The Dilemma of Cosmetic Surgery.* New York, NY: Routledge.

Druss, V. and M.S. Henifin (Eds.). 1979. "Why Are So Many Anorexics Women?" *Women Looking at Biology Looking at Women: A Collection of Feminist Critiques.* Cambridge: Schenkman.

Dull, D. and C. West. 1991. "Accounting for Cosmetic Surgery: The Accomplishment of Gender". *Social Problems* 38: 801-817.

Edgley, Charles and Dennis Brissett. 1990. "Health Nazis and the Cult of the Perfect Body: Some Polemical Observations." *Symbolic Interaction* 13 (2): 257-279.

Elsner, Michael, John F. Galliher and David P. Keys. 1998. "Lindsmith vs. Anslinger: An Early Government Victory in the Failed War on Drugs." *Journal of Criminal Law and Criminology* 88 (2): 661-682.

Ewen, Stuart. 1976. *The Captains of Consciousness.* New York: McGraw-Hill Book Company.

------. 1988. "...Images Without Bottom..." Pp. 47-54 in *The Consumer Society Reader* edited by Juliet B. Schor and Douglas B. Holt. New York, NY: The New Press.

Epstein, Diane and Kathleen Thompson. 1994. *Feeding on Dreams: Why America's Diet Industry Doesn't Work and What Will Work for You.* New York, NY: Macmillan.

Financial News. 2001. "Obesity Experts Highlight Importance of Addressing Obesity and Related Health Consequences; A Call to Action for Increased Obesity Awareness, Prevention and Treatment." *Financial News.* July 24, pp. 23-30. Retrieved February 12, 2003 (http://web.lexisnexis.com/universe/ document?_m=dc055cb2af379de019e111b8ddd678f8&_docnum=28&wchp= dGLbVlb-lSlAl&_md5=dfe8dbdb96b69a87fb243d3145d7968b)

Fiske, John. 1989. "Shopping for Pleasure: Malls, Power, and Resistance." Pp. 306-328 in *The Consumer Society Reader* edited by Juliet B. Schor and Douglas B. Holt. New York, NY: The New Press.

Fowles, Jib. 1996. *Advertising and Popular Culture.* London: Sage Publications.

Friedan, Betty. 1963. "The Sexual Sell." Pp. 26-54 in *The Consumer Society Reader* edited by Juliet B. Schor and Douglas B. Holt. New York, NY: The New Press.

------. 1963. *The Feminine Mystique.* New York, NY: Dell Publishing Company.

Garner, David M., Paul E. Garfinkel, Donald Schwartz, and Michael Thompson. 1980. "Cultural Expectations of Thinness in Women." *Psychological Reports* 47: 483-491.

Gillespie, Marcia Ann. 1993. "Mirror, Mirror." *Essence*, January.

Gimlin, Debra L. 1995. "Cosmetic Surgery: Beauty as Commodity". *Qualitative Sociology* 23: 77-98.

------. 2002. *Body Work: Beauty and Self-Image in American Culture.* Berkeley, CA: University of California Press.

Gladwell, Malcolm. 1998. "The Spin Myth." *The New Yorker.* July, pp. 66-70.

Gorrell, Carin. 2001. "Finding Fault: Magazines May be Abetting-Though Not Aiding-An Epidemic of Eating Disorders." *Psychology Today* 34: 24-26.

Guitierrez, Lisa. 2001. "Herbal Products Promise Women Bust Enlargement." *The Kansas City Star.* February 24, Lifestyle Section K. Retrieved on February 1, 2003 (http://web.lexis-nexis.com/universe/document?_m=b154940ad7ae61b 9623f12750faca685&_docnum=13&wchp=dGLbVlb-lSlAl&_md5=f5c6918 b6c84d6c6ef8aa9dcd45bc3cc).

Hanlon, Michael. 2003. "Can you catch obesity? It is now one of our biggest killers. But is obesity just down to overeating? One scientist believes it is caused by a devastating virus…and we could soon be in the grip of a Fat Plague." *Daily Mail* (London). January 4, pp. 28. Retrieved February 12, 2003 (http://web.lexis-nexis.com/universe/document?_m=dc055cb2af379de019e111b8ddd 678f8&_docnum=33&wchp=dGLbVlb-lSlAl&_md5=cbb50b0bddb513934103 d02ee8c6edf2).

Heiligman, Avron. 1983. "The Incremental Drug Trial in Developing False Doctrine and Its Consequences in the American Drug Scene." *Journal of Sociology and Social Welfare* 4 (1): 19-26.

Hellmich, Nanci. 2002. "Weighing the Cost." *USA Today,* January 21: Life Section, 1D.

Helmer, John. 1975. *Drugs and Minority Oppression.* New York, NY: The Seabury Press.

Herer, Jack. 1998. *The Emperor Has No Clothes: The Authoritative Historical Record of Cannabis and The Conspiracy Against Marijuana.* New York, NY: The AH HA Publishing Co.

Himmelstein, Jerome.1983. *The Strange Career of Marijuana: Politics and Ideology of Drug Control in America.* Westport, CT: Greenwood Press.

------.1987. "From Killer Weed to Drop-Out Drug: The Changing Ideology of Marijuana." *Contemporary Crisis* 7 (1): 13-38.

Kaw, Eugenia. 1993. "Medicalization of Racial Features: Asian-American Women and Cosmetic Surgery." *Medical Anthropology Quarterly* 7: 167-183.

Kemp, Geoffrey. 1998-99. "The Persian Gulf Remains the Strategic Prize." *Survival* 40: 132.

Key, Wilson Brian. 1976. *Media Sexploitation.* New Jersey: NAL Illustrated.

Lamb, Sue C., Lee A. Jackson, Patricia B. Cassiday, and Doris J. Priest. 1993. "Body Figure Preferences of Men and Women: A Comparison of Two Generations." *Sex Roles* 28: 345-358.

Lears, Jackson. 1994. *Fables of Abundance: A Cultural History of Advertising in America.* New York, NY: Basic Books.

Lishak, RS. 1982. "Gray Squirrel Mating Calls: A Spectrographic and Ontogenic Analysis." *Journal of Mammalogy* 63: 661-663.

Litchfield, Rebecca. 2002. "Battery Powered Bra Purports to Increase Bust Size." *University Wire.* November 7. Retrieved on January 28, 2003 (http://web.lexis-nexis.com/universe/document?_m=8cd7f10682066d338292e86c1e19e918&_docnum=27&wchp=dGLbVlb-lSlAl&_md5=d8363e79f668a08c22456b3578c53edf).

Marchand, Roland. 1985. *Advertising the American Dream.* Berkeley, CA: University of California Press.

Marsa, Linda. 2002. "A Tug of War in a Larger Battle; Ephedra is now under intense scrutiny. Its fate could affect other supplements." *Los Angeles Times.* September 2, pp. Home Edition 1. Retrieved on February 19, 2003 (http://web.lexis-nexis.com/universe/document?_m=e79fc707b84949573f3d5c014dfba800&_docnum=12&wchp=dGLbVlb-lSlAl&_md5=8be496e1390b848d6f160adf8f970f22).

Mazur, A. 1986. "U.S. Trends in Feminine Beauty and Overadaptation." *Journal of Sex Research* 22: 281-303.

McKinely, N.M. and J.S. Hyde. 1996. "The Objectified Body Consciousness Scale: Development and Validation." *Psychology of Women Quarterly* 20: 181-215.

Mellican, R. Eugene. 1995. "Breast Implants, the Cult of Beauty, and a Culturally Constructed 'Disease'." *Journal of Popular Culture* 28: 7-17.

Milwaukee Journal Sentinel. 2002. "Company to Stop Selling Breast Enhancing Pills." *Milwaukee Journal Sentinel.* December 31, Final Edition Section pp. 07A. Retrieved on February 23, 2003 (http://web.lexis-nexis.com/universe/document?

_m=4bd88a8c510c31b5c03569747c1cdb10&_docnum=11&wchp=dGLbVlb-lSlAl&_md5=2e076e070766b5ef53fd9db1931af84a).

Minis, Wevonneda A. 2002. "Can Pills Augment Breast Size?" *The Post and Courier* (Charleston, SC). May 13, pp. 1D. Retrieved on February 14, 2003 (http://web.lexis-nexis.com/universe/document?_m=b154940ad7ae61b9623f 12750faca685&_docnum=2&wchp=dGLbVlb-lSlAl&_md5=23e40c2a76e90e 96f23f0bf8db179b80).

Morgan, Kathryn Pauly. 1991. "Women and the Knife: Cosmetic Surgery and the Colonization of Women's Bodies." *Hypatia* 6 (3): 25-53.

Musto, David F. 2000. "Federal Marijuana Laws May Be Going Up In Smoke." *Roanoke Times,* September 17, H24.

Nader, Laura. 1997. "Controlling Processes: Tracing the Dynamic Components of Power." *Current Anthropology* 38: 711-737.

Parloff, Roger. 2003. "Is Fat The Next Tobacco?" *Fortune,* February: 52-69.

Peirce, Kate. 1990. "A Feminist Theoretical Perspective on the Socialization of Teenage Girls Through *Seventeen* Magazine." *Sex Roles* 23 (9-10): 491-500.

Polce-Lynch, Mary, Barbara J. Myers, Wendy Kliewer, and Christopher Kilmartin. 1991. "Adolescent Self-Esteem and Gender: Exploring Relations to Sexual Harassment, Body Image, Media Influence, and Emotional Expression." *Journal of Youth and Adolescence* 30 (2): 225-244.

PR Newswire. 2002. "ConsumerLab.com Finds 'Breast Enhancement' Pills Lack Evidence of Efficacy." *PR Newswire* (Domestic News). April 16. Retrieved on February 25, 2003 (http://web.lexis-nexis.com/universe/document?_m=4bd88a 8c510c31b5c03569747c1cdb10&_docnum=9&wchp=dGLbVlb-lSlAl&_md5= ee6a0bf620ee5828e1e08fdb64459c01).

Pravin, Charlotte. 2002. "Breast Pill Claims 'Rubbish'." *Sunday Star Times* (Auckland, TX). September 22, National Section pp. 3. Retrieved on February 15, 2003 (http://web.lexis-nexis.com/universe/document?_m=4bd88a8c510c31 b5c03569747c1cdb10&_docnum=17&wchp=dGLbVlb-lSlAl&_md5=8012dd 30d672528b08b066afbfef44f2).

Radway, Janice A. 1984. "The Act of Reading Romance: Escape and Instruction." Pp. 169-183 in *The Consumer Society Reader* edited by Juliet B. Schor and Douglas B. Holt. New York, NY: The New Press.

Rana, Elise. 2002. "The Wonder-Bra—Wearing Your Way to Bigger Boobs." *Health Group Media Features*. September 22. Retrieved on February 17, 2003 (http://web.lexis-nexis.com/universe/document?_m=b154940ad7ae61b9623f 12750faca685&_docnum=1&wchp=dGLbVlb-lSlAl&_md5=ba4030a2b4a5fd 7b3efe1a5169cb03a2).

Redfearn, Sue. 2003. "Ephedra Products Thin Out; Braced for the Worst, Makers Sell New Herbs." *Washington Post*. January 14, pp. HEALTH F01. Retrieved on February 19, 2003 (http://web.lexis-nexis.com/universe/ document?_m=e79fc707b84949573f3d5c014dfba800&_docnum=2&wchp= dGLbVlb-lSlAl&_md5=05e98e583de7310f4b94ee55f1ba5877).

Roan, Sheri. 2002. "Problems with ephedra; Controversy over the weight-loss supplement is creating a demand for alternatives. Manufacturers are quick to roll one out, but some experts foresee similar problems." *Los Angeles Times*. December 9, pp. Home Edition 1. Retrieved on February 10, 2003 (http:// web.lexis-nexis.com/universe/document?_m=e79fc707b84949573f3d5c014dfba 800&_docnum=9&wchp=dGLbVlb-lSlAl&_md5=56c2946663225bd2020f96b 48697cfed).

Rock, Paul ed. 1977. *Drugs and Politics*. New Brunswick, NJ: Transaction Books.

Romer, N. 1981. *The Sex-Role Cycle*. New York, NY: Feminist Press.

Roberts, Sally. 2002. "More Employers See Risks, Costs of Obesity; Perception of Disease is Changing." *Business Insurance*, April 22: 41-46.

Robinson, W. 1997. "A Case Study of Globalisation Processes in the Third World: A Transnational Agenda in Nicaragua." *Global Society* 11: 61-91.

Rose, Nikolas. 1990. *Governing the Soul: The Shaping of the Private Self*. New York, NY: Routledge.

Ritzer, George. 1995. *Expressing America*. London: Pine Forge Press.

Salmon, Robert. 1972. "An Analysis of Public Marijuana Policy." *Social Casework* 53, 1: 19-29.

Scanlon, Jennifer. 1995. *Inarticulate Longings: The Ladies Home Journal, Gender, and the Promises of Consumer Culture.* New York, NY: Routledge.

Schor, Juliet. 1998. *The Overspent American.* New York, NY: HarperPerennial.

Sexton, Donald E. and Phyllis Haberman. 1974. "Women in Magazine Advertisements." *Journal of Advertising Research* 14 (4): 41-46.

Silverstein, Brett, V. Perdue, Barbara Peterson, and Eileen Kelly. 1986. "The Role of the Mass Media in Promoting a Thin Standard of Bodily Attractiveness for Women." *Sex Roles* 14: 519-532.

Sinclair, Jon. 1987. *Images Incorporated.* New York, NY: Croom Helm Publishing.

Spencer, William J. 2000. "Appropriating Cultural Discourses: Notes on a Framework for Constructionist Analyses of the Language of Claims-Making." *Perspectives on Social Problems* 12: 25-40.

Spillman, Diana Marie and Caroline Everington. 1989. "Somatotypes Revisited: Have the Media Changed Our Perception of the Female Body Image?" *Psychological Reports* 64: 887-890.

Stokes, DL and P Dee Boersma. 2000. "Nesting Density and Reproductive Success in a Colonial Seabird, the Magellanic Penguin." *Ecology* 81: 2878-2891.

Sullivan, Deborah. 1993. "Cosmetic Surgery: The Cutting Edge of Commercial Medicine." *Research in the Sociology of Health Care* 10: 97-115.

Sullivan, Patrick F., Cynthia M. Bulik, Frances A. Carter, Kelly A. Gendall, and Peter R. Joyce. 1996. "The Significance of a Prior History of Anorexia in Bulimia Nervosa." *International Journal of Eating Disorders* 20: 253-261.

Tong, Rosemarie Putnam. 1998. *Feminist Thought.* Boulder, CO: Westview Press.

Torrens, Kathleen M. 1998. "I Can Get Any Job and Feel Like a Butterfly! Symbolic Violence in the TV Advertising of Jenny Craig." *Journal of Communication Inquiry* 22: 27-42.

Turner, Sherry. 1997. "The Influence of Fashion Magazines on the Body Image Satisfaction of College Women: An Exploratory Analysis." *Adolescence* 32: 603-614.

University Wire. 2001. "Experts Address Obesity and Health Related Problems." *Expanded Reporting*. August 25, pp. 17-18. Retrieved on February 5, 2003 (http://web.lexis-nexis.com/universe/document?_m=dc055cb2af379de019e111b 8ddd678f8&_docnum=47&wchp=dGLbVlb-lSlAl&_md5=03f729672e424bdd 8e5db409f3ff028a).

Wolf, Naomi. 1991. *The Beauty Myth*. New York, NY: William Morrow and Co., Inc.

www.dexatrim.com

www.jennycraig.com/programs/faq-pi.asp

www.magazine.org/resources/fact_sheets.html.

www.metabolife.com

www.metabolife.com/about/history.htm

www.naaso.org

www.naturalfirm.com

www.naturalbreast.com

www.obesity.org

www.plasticsurgery.org

www.plasticsurgery.org/mediactr/2001_expanded_stats/average_surgeons.pdf

www.smallbreastsolutions.com

www.weightwatchers.com

www.wellquestintl.com

0-595-35017-8

www.ingramcontent.com/pod-product-compliance
Lightning Source LLC
Chambersburg PA
CBHW030407290526
45785CB00004B/1929